Welcome to ***"Ramen Cookbook for Teens: 115+ Homemade Ramen Favorites Every Teen Can Cook."*** Whether you're new to cooking or already enjoy experimenting in the kitchen, this cookbook is your passport to a world of delicious and creative ramen dishes that are easy to prepare and sure to impress.

Why Ramen?

Ramen has captured the hearts and taste buds of people around the world for its comforting noodles, savory broths, and endless variations. In this cookbook, we celebrate the versatility of ramen and show you how to create homemade versions that are healthier, more flavorful, and tailored to your preferences.

What You'll Find in This Book

This cookbook is packed with over 115 recipes that range from classic ramen bowls to innovative twists and adaptations. Each recipe is designed with teens in mind, emphasizing simplicity, accessibility, and fun. Whether you're craving a quick weeknight meal, planning a gathering with friends, or looking to impress your family, you'll find plenty of options to suit every occasion.

Key Features:

- ***Easy-to-Follow Recipes:*** Step-by-step instructions and helpful tips make it easy for teens to confidently prepare delicious ramen dishes at home.

- ***Variety and Creativity:*** Explore a wide range of flavors, ingredients, and techniques to create your own personalized ramen bowls.

- ***Nutritious and Balanced:*** Discover how homemade ramen can be both satisfying and nutritious with fresh ingredients and flavorful broths.

- ***Tips and Tricks:*** Learn essential cooking skills, ingredient substitutions, and ways to customize recipes to suit your taste preferences.

Benefits of Cooking Ramen:

Cooking ramen at home offers numerous benefits beyond just a delicious meal:

- ***Skill Development:*** Enhance your cooking skills and gain confidence in the kitchen.

- ***Healthier Options:*** Control over ingredients allows you to create healthier versions of your favorite ramen dishes.

- ***Creativity and Expression:*** Experiment with flavors and ingredients to develop your own signature ramen creations.

- ***Family and Friends:*** Share your love of cooking by preparing homemade meals that bring people together.

Get ready to embark on a delicious adventure with ***"Ramen Cookbook for Teens: 115+ Homemade Ramen Favorites Every Teen Can Cook."*** Let's dive in, get cooking, and discover the joy of creating flavorful and satisfying ramen bowls that will become your new favorites.

1. Classic Shoyu Ramen

Ingredient:
- 6 cups chicken or vegetable broth
- 2 tablespoons soy sauce
- 1 tablespoon mirin
- 1 teaspoon sesame oil
- 1 garlic clove, minced
- 1·inch piece fresh ginger, peeled and grated
- 8 oz ramen noodles
- 2 soft·boiled eggs, halved
- 1 cup shredded cooked chicken or pork (optional)
- 1 cup sliced mushrooms
- 1 cup shredded cabbage or spinach
- Sliced green onions, for garnish

Instructions:
1. In a large pot, combine the broth, soy sauce, mirin, sesame oil, garlic, and ginger. Bring to a simmer over medium heat.

2. Add the ramen noodles and cook according to package instructions, usually 2·3 minutes.

3. Divide the noodles and broth between 4 bowls. Top each bowl with a soft·boiled egg, shredded meat (if using), mushrooms, and cabbage or spinach. Garnish with sliced green onions.

This ramen is flavorful but not too spicy, making it a great option for teens. The soft·boiled egg adds protein and richness, while the vegetables provide nutrients. Feel free to customize the toppings to your liking.

2. Spicy Miso Ramen

Ingredient:

• 6 cups chicken or vegetable broth
• 3 tablespoons miso paste (white or yellow)
• 1 tablespoon sriracha or other hot sauce
• 1 tablespoon brown sugar
• 1 teaspoon sesame oil
• 1 garlic clove, minced
• 1•inch piece fresh ginger, peeled and grated
• 8 oz ramen noodles
• 2 soft•boiled eggs, halved
• 1 cup sliced mushrooms
• 1 cup shredded carrots
• 1 cup baby spinach or chopped kale
• Sliced green onions, for garnish
• Toasted sesame seeds, for garnish

Instructions:

1. In a large pot, whisk together the broth, miso paste, sriracha, brown sugar, sesame oil, garlic, and ginger. Bring to a simmer over medium heat.

2. Add the ramen noodles and cook according to package instructions, usually 2•3 minutes.

3. Divide the noodles and broth between 4 bowls. Top each bowl with a soft•boiled egg, mushrooms, carrots, and spinach or kale.

4. Garnish with sliced green onions and toasted sesame seeds.

This ramen has a nice kick of spice from the sriracha, balanced by the sweetness of the brown sugar. The miso paste adds a savory umami flavor. The soft•boiled egg, vegetables, and protein•rich noodles make this a nutritious and filling meal for teens.

3. Tonkotsu Ramen

Ingredient:

- 1 lb pork bones (neck bones or trotters)
- 1 onion, chopped
- 3 garlic cloves, minced
- 1·inch piece fresh ginger, peeled and sliced
- 8 cups water
- 2 tablespoons soy sauce
- 1 tablespoon mirin
- 1 teaspoon salt
- 8 oz ramen noodles
- 2 soft·boiled eggs, halved
- 1 cup sliced pork belly or chashu pork
- 1 cup sliced mushrooms
- 1 cup bean sprouts
- Sliced green onions, for garnish
- Toasted sesame seeds, for garnish

Instructions:

1. In a large pot, combine the pork bones, onion, garlic, and ginger. Add the water and bring to a boil over high heat.

2. Reduce heat to medium·low and simmer for 6·8 hours, skimming any scum that rises to the surface. The broth should become rich and creamy.

3. Strain the broth through a fine·mesh sieve, discarding the solids. Return the broth to the pot and stir in the soy sauce, mirin, and salt.

4. Bring the broth back to a simmer. Add the ramen noodles and cook according to package instructions, usually 2·3 minutes.

5. Divide the noodles and broth between 4 bowls. Top each bowl with a soft·boiled egg, sliced pork, mushrooms, and bean sprouts.

6. Garnish with sliced green onions and toasted sesame seeds.

Tonkotsu ramen features a rich, creamy pork bone broth that is simmered for hours to extract maximum flavor. The soft·boiled egg, tender pork, and fresh vegetables make this a hearty and satisfying meal for teens.

4. Shio Ramen

Ingredient:

- 6 cups chicken or vegetable broth
- 2 tablespoons salt
- 1 tablespoon mirin
- 1 teaspoon sesame oil
- 1 garlic clove, minced
- 1·inch piece fresh ginger, peeled and grated
- 8 oz ramen noodles
- 2 soft·boiled eggs, halved
- 1 cup sliced roasted chicken or pork (optional)
- 1 cup sliced mushrooms
- 1 cup shredded cabbage or spinach
- Sliced green onions, for garnish
- Toasted sesame seeds, for garnish

Instructions:

1. In a large pot, combine the broth, salt, mirin, sesame oil, garlic, and ginger. Bring to a simmer over medium heat.

2. Add the ramen noodles and cook according to package instructions, usually 2·3 minutes.

3. Divide the noodles and broth between 4 bowls. Top each bowl with a soft·boiled egg, sliced meat (if using), mushrooms, and cabbage or spinach.

4. Garnish with sliced green onions and toasted sesame seeds.

Shio ramen features a simple, yet flavorful broth seasoned with salt. The soft·boiled egg and tender meat or vegetables make this a satisfying and nutritious meal for teens. The garnishes add a nice crunch and flavor contrast.

This version is lighter and less intense than some other ramen styles, making it a great option for younger eaters. Feel free to adjust the salt level to your taste.

5. Vegetarian Ramen

Ingredient:

• 6 cups vegetable broth
• 2 tablespoons miso paste
• 1 tablespoon soy sauce
• 1 teaspoon sesame oil
• 1 garlic clove, minced
• 1•inch piece fresh ginger, peeled and grated
• 8 oz ramen noodles
• 1 block firm tofu, cubed
• 1 cup sliced mushrooms
• 1 cup shredded carrots
• 1 cup baby spinach or chopped kale
• Sliced green onions, for garnish
• Toasted sesame seeds, for garnish

Instructions:

1. In a large pot, whisk together the vegetable broth, miso paste, soy sauce, sesame oil, garlic, and ginger. Bring to a simmer over medium heat.

2. Add the ramen noodles and cook according to package instructions, usually 2•3 minutes.

3. Divide the noodles and broth between 4 bowls. Top each bowl with cubed tofu, sliced mushrooms, shredded carrots, and baby spinach or kale.

4. Garnish with sliced green onions and toasted sesame seeds.

This vegetarian ramen is packed with flavor from the miso, soy sauce, and aromatic ginger and garlic. The tofu provides plant•based protein, while the vegetables add nutrients and fiber.

The ramen noodles make this a hearty and satisfying meal for teens. Feel free to adjust the vegetables to your liking or add other toppings like boiled eggs or crispy tofu.

6. Chicken Ramen

Ingredient:

• 6 cups chicken broth
• 2 tablespoons soy sauce
• 1 tablespoon mirin
• 1 teaspoon sesame oil
• 1 garlic clove, minced
• 1•inch piece fresh ginger, peeled and grated
• 8 oz ramen noodles
• 2 cups shredded cooked chicken
• 1 cup sliced mushrooms
• 1 cup shredded carrots
• 1 cup baby spinach or chopped kale
• Sliced green onions, for garnish
• Soft•boiled eggs (optional)

Instructions:

1. In a large pot, combine the chicken broth, soy sauce, mirin, sesame oil, garlic, and ginger. Bring to a simmer over medium heat.

2. Add the ramen noodles and cook according to package instructions, usually 2•3 minutes.

3. Divide the noodles and broth between 4 bowls. Top each bowl with shredded chicken, sliced mushrooms, shredded carrots, and baby spinach or kale.

4. Garnish with sliced green onions. You can also top with soft•boiled eggs, if desired.

This chicken ramen is a simple yet flavorful option that teens are sure to enjoy. The shredded chicken adds protein, while the vegetables provide nutrients. The broth is seasoned with soy sauce, mirin, and aromatic garlic and ginger.

Feel free to adjust the toppings to your liking or add other ingredients like corn, bean sprouts, or crispy fried onions. This is a versatile and customizable ramen dish.

7. Beef Ramen

Ingredient:

• 6 cups beef or chicken broth
• 2 tablespoons soy sauce
• 1 tablespoon mirin
• 1 teaspoon sesame oil
• 1 garlic clove, minced
• 1•inch piece fresh ginger, peeled and grated
• 8 oz ramen noodles
• 1 lb thinly sliced beef (such as sirloin or flank steak)
• 1 cup sliced mushrooms
• 1 cup shredded carrots
• 1 cup baby spinach or chopped kale
• Sliced green onions, for garnish
• Soft•boiled eggs (optional)

Instructions:

1. In a large pot, combine the broth, soy sauce, mirin, sesame oil, garlic, and ginger. Bring to a simmer over medium heat.

2. Add the ramen noodles and cook according to package instructions, usually 2•3 minutes.

3. Add the sliced beef to the simmering broth and cook for 2•3 minutes, until the beef is cooked through.

4. Divide the noodles, broth, and beef between 4 bowls. Top each bowl with sliced mushrooms, shredded carrots, and baby spinach or kale.

5. Garnish with sliced green onions. You can also top with soft•boiled eggs, if desired.

This beef ramen is a hearty and satisfying option for teens. The thinly sliced beef cooks quickly in the hot broth, making it a simple and easy•to•prepare meal. The vegetables add nutrition and color.

Feel free to adjust the amount of beef or swap in a different protein, such as chicken or tofu, based on your preferences. This recipe is easily customizable to suit individual tastes.

8. Pork Ramen

Ingredient:

- 6 cups chicken or pork broth
- 2 tablespoons soy sauce
- 1 tablespoon mirin
- 1 teaspoon sesame oil
- 1 garlic clove, minced
- 1·inch piece fresh ginger, peeled and grated
- 8 oz ramen noodles
- 1 lb thinly sliced pork (such as pork loin or pork belly)
- 1 cup sliced mushrooms
- 1 cup shredded cabbage or spinach
- 2 soft·boiled eggs, halved (optional)
- Sliced green onions, for garnish
- Toasted sesame seeds, for garnish

Instructions:

1. In a large pot, combine the broth, soy sauce, mirin, sesame oil, garlic, and ginger. Bring to a simmer over medium heat.

2. Add the ramen noodles and cook according to package instructions, usually 2·3 minutes.

3. Add the sliced pork to the simmering broth and cook for 2·3 minutes, until the pork is cooked through.

4. Divide the noodles, broth, and pork between 4 bowls. Top each bowl with sliced mushrooms, shredded cabbage or spinach, and soft·boiled eggs (if using).

5. Garnish with sliced green onions and toasted sesame seeds.

This pork ramen features tender, flavorful pork that cooks quickly in the hot broth. The mushrooms, cabbage or spinach, and soft·boiled egg (if using) add nutrition and texture.

The broth is seasoned with soy sauce, mirin, and aromatic garlic and ginger, giving it a savory, umami·rich flavor. This is a hearty and satisfying ramen dish that teens are sure to enjoy.

Feel free to adjust the protein, vegetables, or other toppings to your liking.

9. Seafood Ramen

Ingredient:

- 6 cups seafood or chicken broth
- 2 tablespoons miso paste
- 1 tablespoon soy sauce
- 1 teaspoon sesame oil
- 1 garlic clove, minced
- 1·inch piece fresh ginger, peeled and grated
- 8 oz ramen noodles
- 1 lb mixed seafood (such as shrimp, scallops, and squid), chopped
- 1 cup sliced mushrooms
- 1 cup shredded carrots
- 1 cup baby spinach or chopped kale
- Sliced green onions, for garnish
- Lime wedges, for serving

Instructions:

1. In a large pot, whisk together the seafood or chicken broth, miso paste, soy sauce, sesame oil, garlic, and ginger. Bring to a simmer over medium heat.

2. Add the ramen noodles and cook according to package instructions, usually 2·3 minutes.

3. Add the chopped seafood to the simmering broth and cook for 2·3 minutes, until the seafood is cooked through.

4. Divide the noodles, broth, and seafood between 4 bowls. Top each bowl with sliced mushrooms, shredded carrots, and baby spinach or kale. Garnish with sliced green onions and serve with lime wedges on the side.

This seafood ramen is a delicious and nutritious option for teens. The broth is flavored with savory miso paste and aromatic garlic and ginger, while the mixed seafood provides a variety of textures and flavors.

The vegetables add color, crunch, and extra nutrients. The lime wedges provide a bright, acidic contrast to the rich broth.

Feel free to adjust the types of seafood used or swap in other proteins, such as chicken or tofu, based on your preferences.

10. Miso Butter Corn Ramen

Ingredient:

• 6 cups chicken or vegetable broth
• 2 tablespoons white or yellow miso paste
• 2 tablespoons unsalted butter
• 1 cup frozen corn kernels
• 1 garlic clove, minced
• 1·inch piece fresh ginger, peeled and grated
• 8 oz ramen noodles
• 1 cup shredded cooked chicken or tofu
• 1 cup sliced mushrooms
• 1 cup baby spinach or chopped kale
• Sliced green onions, for garnish
• Toasted sesame seeds, for garnish

Instructions:

1. In a large pot, whisk together the broth and miso paste until the miso is fully dissolved.

2. Add the butter, frozen corn, garlic, and ginger. Bring the mixture to a simmer over medium heat, stirring occasionally, until the butter is melted and the corn is heated through, about 5 minutes.

3. Add the ramen noodles and cook according to package instructions, usually 2·3 minutes.

4. Stir in the shredded chicken or tofu, sliced mushrooms, and baby spinach or kale. Cook for an additional 1·2 minutes until the greens are wilted.

5. Divide the noodles, broth, and toppings between 4 bowls.

6. Garnish with sliced green onions and toasted sesame seeds.

This miso butter corn ramen has a rich, creamy broth that's flavored with savory miso and sweet corn. The butter adds a luxurious mouthfeel.

The shredded chicken or tofu, mushrooms, and greens provide protein, fiber, and nutrients, making this a well·balanced and satisfying meal for teens. The garnishes add freshness and crunch.

11. Cheesy Ramen

Ingredient:

- 6 cups chicken or vegetable broth
- 2 tablespoons unsalted butter
- 2 tablespoons all•purpose flour
- 1 cup shredded cheddar cheese
- 1/2 cup grated Parmesan cheese
- 1 teaspoon garlic powder
- 1/2 teaspoon onion powder
- 1/4 teaspoon cayenne pepper (optional)
- 8 oz ramen noodles
- 1 cup cooked shredded chicken or crumbled tofu (optional)
- 1 cup frozen peas
- Sliced green onions, for garnish

Instructions:

1. In a large pot, bring the broth to a simmer over medium heat.

2. In a separate saucepan, melt the butter over medium heat. Whisk in the flour and cook for 1•2 minutes to make a roux.

3. Gradually whisk the hot broth into the roux until smooth and thickened, about 2•3 minutes.

4. Remove the pot from heat and stir in the cheddar cheese, Parmesan cheese, garlic powder, onion powder, and cayenne pepper (if using) until the cheese is melted and the sauce is smooth.

5. Add the ramen noodles and cook according to package instructions, usually 2•3 minutes.

6. Stir in the cooked chicken or tofu (if using) and frozen peas. Cook for an additional 1•2 minutes until heated through. Divide the cheesy ramen between 4 bowls and garnish with sliced green onions.

This cheesy ramen is a comforting and indulgent twist on classic ramen. The creamy, cheese•based broth is flavored with garlic, onion, and a touch of heat from the cayenne.

The addition of chicken or tofu and peas makes this a more substantial and nutritious meal for teens. The green onions provide a fresh contrast to the rich, cheesy broth.

12. Kimchi Ramen

Ingredient:

- 6 cups chicken or vegetable broth
- 1/2 cup kimchi, chopped, plus more for serving
- 2 tablespoons gochujang (Korean chili paste)
- 1 tablespoon soy sauce
- 1 teaspoon sesame oil
- 1 garlic clove, minced
- 1·inch piece fresh ginger, peeled and grated
- 8 oz ramen noodles
- 1 cup shredded cooked chicken or tofu
- 1 cup sliced mushrooms
- 1 cup shredded cabbage or spinach
- Sliced green onions, for garnish
- Sesame seeds, for garnish

Instructions:

1. In a large pot, combine the broth, chopped kimchi, gochujang, soy sauce, sesame oil, garlic, and ginger. Bring to a simmer over medium heat.

2. Add the ramen noodles and cook according to package instructions, usually 2·3 minutes.

3. Stir in the shredded chicken or tofu, sliced mushrooms, and shredded cabbage or spinach. Cook for an additional 1·2 minutes until the greens are wilted.

4. Divide the noodles, broth, and toppings between 4 bowls.

5. Garnish with additional chopped kimchi, sliced green onions, and sesame seeds.

This kimchi ramen features a spicy, flavorful broth made with gochujang (Korean chili paste) and kimchi. The kimchi adds a tangy, fermented flavor that pairs well with the savory broth.

The shredded chicken or tofu, mushrooms, and greens provide protein, fiber, and nutrients, making this a well·rounded meal for teens. The garnishes of green onions and sesame seeds add freshness and crunch.

Feel free to adjust the amount of gochujang or kimchi to suit your spice preference. You can also add other toppings like soft·boiled eggs or crispy fried onions.

13. BBQ Ramen

Ingredient:

• 6 cups chicken or beef broth
• 1/2 cup barbecue sauce
• 2 tablespoons soy sauce
• 1 tablespoon brown sugar
• 1 teaspoon smoked paprika
• 1 garlic clove, minced
• 8 oz ramen noodles
• 1 lb pulled pork or shredded chicken
• 1 cup sliced mushrooms
• 1 cup shredded cabbage or coleslaw mix
• Sliced green onions, for garnish
• Crushed peanuts or toasted sesame seeds, for garnish

Instructions:

1. In a large pot, combine the broth, barbecue sauce, soy sauce, brown sugar, smoked paprika, and garlic. Bring to a simmer over medium heat.

2. Add the ramen noodles and cook according to package instructions, usually 2•3 minutes.

3. Stir in the pulled pork or shredded chicken, sliced mushrooms, and shredded cabbage or coleslaw mix. Cook for an additional 1•2 minutes until heated through.

4. Divide the noodles, broth, and toppings between 4 bowls.

5. Garnish with sliced green onions and crushed peanuts or toasted sesame seeds.

This BBQ ramen puts a delicious twist on classic ramen. The broth is infused with the sweet and smoky flavors of barbecue sauce, soy sauce, and smoked paprika.

The pulled pork or shredded chicken adds heartiness, while the mushrooms and cabbage provide crunch and freshness. The green onions and peanuts or sesame seeds add a nice finishing touch.

This ramen dish is sure to be a hit with teens, as it combines familiar barbecue flavors with the comforting noodles and broth of ramen.Feel free to adjust the amount of barbecue sauce or other seasonings to suit your taste preferences.

14. Thai Curry Ramen

Ingredient:

- 6 cups chicken or vegetable broth
- 1/2 cup coconut milk
- 2 tablespoons red curry paste
- 1 tablespoon fish sauce
- 1 tablespoon brown sugar
- 1 garlic clove, minced
- 1•inch piece fresh ginger, peeled and grated
- 8 oz ramen noodles
- 1 cup sliced chicken or tofu
- 1 cup sliced mushrooms
- 1 cup shredded carrots
- 1 cup baby spinach or chopped kale
- Sliced green onions, for garnish
- Chopped cilantro, for garnish
- Lime wedges, for serving

Instructions:

1. In a large pot, combine the broth, coconut milk, red curry paste, fish sauce, brown sugar, garlic, and ginger. Bring to a simmer over medium heat.

2. Add the ramen noodles and cook according to package instructions, usually 2•3 minutes.

3. Stir in the sliced chicken or tofu, mushrooms, carrots, and baby spinach or kale. Cook for an additional 2•3 minutes until the protein is cooked through and the vegetables are tender.

4. Divide the noodles, broth, and toppings between 4 bowls.

5. Garnish with sliced green onions and chopped cilantro. Serve with lime wedges on the side.

This Thai curry ramen features a rich, creamy broth infused with the bold flavors of red curry paste, coconut milk, fish sauce, and brown sugar. The ginger and garlic add aromatic depth.

The sliced chicken or tofu, mushrooms, carrots, and greens provide a variety of textures and nutrients. The fresh garnishes of green onions and cilantro, along with the lime wedges, help to balance the bold curry flavors.

This ramen dish is a great way to introduce teens to the vibrant tastes of Thai cuisine in a comforting, noodle•based format. Feel free to adjust the amount of curry paste or other seasonings to suit your spice preference.

15. Coconut Lime Ramen

Ingredient:

- 4 cups chicken or vegetable broth
- 1 (13.5 oz) can coconut milk
- 2 tablespoons lime juice
- 1 tablespoon fish sauce
- 1 tablespoon brown sugar
- 1 teaspoon red curry paste
- 1 garlic clove, minced
- 1•inch piece fresh ginger, peeled and grated
- 8 oz ramen noodles

- 1 cup shredded cooked chicken or tofu
- 1 cup sliced mushrooms
- 1 cup shredded carrots
- 1 cup bean sprouts
- Sliced green onions, for garnish
- Chopped cilantro, for garnish
- Lime wedges, for serving

Instructions:

1. In a large pot, combine the broth, coconut milk, lime juice, fish sauce, brown sugar, curry paste, garlic, and ginger. Bring to a simmer over medium heat.

2. Add the ramen noodles and cook according to package instructions, usually 2•3 minutes.

3. Stir in the shredded chicken or tofu, mushrooms, carrots, and bean sprouts. Cook for an additional 2•3 minutes.

4. Divide the noodles, broth, and toppings between 4 bowls.

5. Garnish with sliced green onions and chopped cilantro. Serve with lime wedges on the side.

This coconut lime ramen has a unique and flavorful broth that combines the richness of coconut milk with the bright acidity of lime and the savory depth of fish sauce. The red curry paste adds a subtle heat.

The shredded chicken or tofu, vegetables, and ramen noodles make this a hearty and satisfying meal for teens. The fresh garnishes of green onions and cilantro provide a nice contrast. Feel free to adjust the amount of curry paste or other seasonings to suit your taste preferences.

16. Sriracha Ramen

Ingredient:

- 6 cups chicken or vegetable broth
- 3 tablespoons sriracha (or more to taste)
- 2 tablespoons soy sauce
- 1 tablespoon brown sugar
- 1 teaspoon sesame oil
- 1 garlic clove, minced
- 1-inch piece fresh ginger, peeled and grated
- 8 oz ramen noodles
- 1 cup shredded cooked chicken or tofu
- 1 cup sliced mushrooms
- 1 cup shredded carrots
- 1 cup baby spinach or chopped kale
- Sliced green onions, for garnish
- Crushed peanuts or sesame seeds, for garnish

Instructions:

1. In a large pot, combine the broth, sriracha, soy sauce, brown sugar, sesame oil, garlic, and ginger. Bring to a simmer over medium heat.

2. Add the ramen noodles and cook according to package instructions, usually 2-3 minutes.

3. Stir in the shredded chicken or tofu, sliced mushrooms, shredded carrots, and baby spinach or kale. Cook for an additional 1-2 minutes until the greens are wilted.

4. Divide the noodles, broth, and toppings between 4 bowls. Garnish with sliced green onions and crushed peanuts or sesame seeds.

This sriracha ramen packs a flavorful punch with the addition of the spicy, tangy sriracha sauce. The brown sugar and sesame oil help to balance the heat and add depth of flavor.

The shredded chicken or tofu, mushrooms, carrots, and greens provide a nutritious and filling meal for teens. The crunchy garnishes of green onions and peanuts or sesame seeds add a nice textural contrast.

Feel free to adjust the amount of sriracha to your desired spice level. You can also add other toppings like soft-boiled eggs or crispy fried onions.

17. Garlic Parmesan Ramen

Ingredient:

• 6 cups chicken or vegetable broth
• 3 garlic cloves, minced
• 1/2 cup grated Parmesan cheese
• 2 tablespoons butter
• 1 tablespoon lemon juice
• 1 teaspoon dried oregano
• 1/4 teaspoon red pepper flakes (optional)
• 8 oz ramen noodles
• 1 cup shredded cooked chicken or tofu
• 1 cup sliced mushrooms
• 1 cup baby spinach or arugula
• Sliced green onions, for garnish
• Freshly cracked black pepper, for serving

Instructions:

1. In a large pot, bring the broth to a simmer over medium heat. Add the minced garlic and cook for 1•2 minutes until fragrant.

2. Reduce the heat to low and stir in the Parmesan cheese, butter, lemon juice, oregano, and red pepper flakes (if using). Whisk until the cheese is melted and the sauce is smooth.

3. Add the ramen noodles and cook according to package instructions, usually 2•3 minutes.

4. Stir in the shredded chicken or tofu, sliced mushrooms, and baby spinach or arugula. Cook for an additional 1•2 minutes until the greens are wilted.

5. Divide the noodles, broth, and toppings between 4 bowls. Garnish with sliced green onions and freshly cracked black pepper.

This garlic Parmesan ramen has a rich, creamy broth that's infused with the savory flavors of garlic, Parmesan, and oregano. The lemon juice adds a bright, tangy note.

The shredded chicken or tofu, mushrooms, and greens provide protein, fiber, and nutrients, making this a well•rounded meal for teens. The green onions and black pepper add freshness and a touch of heat. Feel free to adjust the amount of Parmesan or red pepper flakes to suit your taste preferences.

18. Spicy Peanut Butter Ramen

Ingredient:

• 6 cups chicken or vegetable broth
• 1/2 cup creamy peanut butter
• 2 tablespoons soy sauce
• 2 tablespoons sriracha (or more to taste)
• 1 tablespoon brown sugar
• 1 teaspoon sesame oil
• 1 garlic clove, minced
• 1•inch piece fresh ginger, peeled and grated
• 8 oz ramen noodles
• 1 cup shredded cooked chicken or tofu
• 1 cup sliced mushrooms
• 1 cup shredded carrots
• 1 cup baby spinach or chopped kale
• Sliced green onions, for garnish
• Chopped peanuts, for garnish

Instructions:

1. In a large pot, whisk together the broth, peanut butter, soy sauce, sriracha, brown sugar, sesame oil, garlic, and ginger. Bring to a simmer over medium heat.

2. Add the ramen noodles and cook according to package instructions, usually 2•3 minutes.

3. Stir in the shredded chicken or tofu, sliced mushrooms, shredded carrots, and baby spinach or kale. Cook for an additional 1•2 minutes until the greens are wilted.

4. Divide the noodles, broth, and toppings between 4 bowls. Garnish with sliced green onions and chopped peanuts.

This spicy peanut butter ramen has a rich, creamy broth that's infused with the nutty flavor of peanut butter and the heat of sriracha. The brown sugar and sesame oil help to balance the flavors.

The shredded chicken or tofu, mushrooms, carrots, and greens provide a nutritious and filling meal for teens. The crunchy garnishes of green onions and peanuts add a nice textural contrast.

Feel free to adjust the amount of sriracha to your desired spice level. You can also add other toppings like crushed red pepper flakes or chopped cilantro.

19. Buffalo Chicken Ramen

Ingredient:

- 6 cups chicken broth
- 1/2 cup buffalo sauce (such as Frank's RedHot)
- 2 tablespoons unsalted butter
- 1 tablespoon soy sauce
- 1 teaspoon garlic powder
- 1/2 teaspoon onion powder
- 8 oz ramen noodles
- 2 cups shredded cooked chicken
- 1 cup sliced celery
- 1 cup shredded carrots
- 1 cup crumbled blue cheese (optional)
- Sliced green onions, for garnish

Instructions:

1. In a large pot, combine the chicken broth, buffalo sauce, butter, soy sauce, garlic powder, and onion powder. Bring to a simmer over medium heat, stirring occasionally, until the butter is melted and the flavors are blended.

2. Add the ramen noodles and cook according to package instructions, usually 2•3 minutes.

3. Stir in the shredded chicken, sliced celery, and shredded carrots. Cook for an additional 1•2 minutes until heated through.

4. Divide the buffalo chicken ramen between 4 bowls.

5. Top each bowl with crumbled blue cheese (if using) and sliced green onions.

This buffalo chicken ramen combines the bold, spicy flavors of buffalo sauce with the comforting noodles and broth of ramen. The shredded chicken, celery, and carrots add protein, fiber, and nutrients.

The optional blue cheese topping provides a creamy, tangy contrast to the heat of the buffalo sauce. The green onions add a fresh, crunchy garnish.

This ramen dish is sure to be a hit with teens who enjoy the flavors of buffalo chicken. Feel free to adjust the amount of buffalo sauce to suit your spice preference.

20. Creamy Alfredo Ramen

Ingredient:

- 6 cups chicken or vegetable broth
- 1/2 cup heavy cream
- 1/2 cup grated Parmesan cheese
- 2 tablespoons unsalted butter
- 1 garlic clove, minced
- 1/4 teaspoon ground black pepper
- 8 oz ramen noodles
- 1 cup cooked shredded chicken or tofu
- 1 cup sliced mushrooms
- 1 cup baby spinach or chopped kale
- Chopped parsley, for garnish

Instructions:

1. In a large pot, combine the broth, heavy cream, Parmesan cheese, butter, garlic, and black pepper. Bring to a simmer over medium heat, stirring occasionally, until the cheese is melted and the sauce is smooth.

2. Add the ramen noodles and cook according to package instructions, usually 2·3 minutes.

3. Stir in the cooked shredded chicken or tofu, sliced mushrooms, and baby spinach or kale. Cook for an additional 1·2 minutes until the greens are wilted.

4. Divide the creamy alfredo ramen between 4 bowls.

5. Garnish with chopped parsley.

This creamy alfredo ramen puts a decadent spin on classic ramen. The rich, creamy sauce is made with heavy cream, Parmesan cheese, and a touch of garlic, creating a luxurious broth.

The shredded chicken or tofu, mushrooms, and greens add protein, fiber, and nutrients to make this a well·rounded meal for teens. The parsley garnish provides a fresh, herbal note.

This ramen dish is sure to be a hit with teens who enjoy creamy, comforting flavors. Feel free to adjust the amount of Parmesan or add other toppings like roasted vegetables or crispy bacon.

21. Low•Sodium Ramen

Ingredient:

• 6 cups low•sodium chicken or vegetable broth
• 1 tablespoon low•sodium soy sauce
• 1 teaspoon mirin
• 1/2 teaspoon sesame oil
• 1 garlic clove, minced
• 1•inch piece fresh ginger, peeled and grated
• 8 oz low•sodium ramen noodles
• 1 cup sliced mushrooms
• 1 cup shredded cooked chicken or tofu
• 1 cup shredded cabbage or spinach
• Sliced green onions, for garnish
• Soft•boiled egg (optional)

Instructions:

1. In a large pot, combine the low•sodium broth, soy sauce, mirin, sesame oil, garlic, and ginger. Bring to a simmer over medium heat.

2. Add the low•sodium ramen noodles and cook according to package instructions, usually 2•3 minutes.

3. Stir in the sliced mushrooms, shredded chicken or tofu, and shredded cabbage or spinach. Cook for an additional 2•3 minutes.

4. Divide the noodles, broth, and toppings between 4 bowls.

5. Garnish with sliced green onions. You can also top with a soft•boiled egg, if desired.

This low•sodium ramen is a healthier option that still delivers on flavor. By using low•sodium broth and soy sauce, as well as low•sodium ramen noodles, the overall sodium content is significantly reduced.

The mushrooms, chicken or tofu, and greens provide protein, fiber, and nutrients, making this a balanced and satisfying meal for teens. The garnishes add freshness and crunch.

Feel free to adjust the specific ingredients or toppings to your liking. This recipe can be easily customized to suit individual preferences.

22. Vegetable Ramen

Ingredient:

• 6 cups vegetable broth
• 2 tablespoons miso paste
• 1 tablespoon soy sauce
• 1 teaspoon sesame oil
• 1 garlic clove, minced
• 1•inch piece fresh ginger, peeled and grated
• 8 oz ramen noodles
• 1 cup sliced mushrooms
• 1 cup shredded carrots
• 1 cup broccoli florets
• 1 cup baby bok choy, chopped
• 1 cup cubed firm tofu
• Sliced green onions, for garnish
• Toasted sesame seeds, for garnish

Instructions:

1. In a large pot, whisk together the vegetable broth, miso paste, soy sauce, sesame oil, garlic, and ginger. Bring to a simmer over medium heat.

2. Add the ramen noodles and cook according to package instructions, usually 2•3 minutes.

3. Stir in the sliced mushrooms, shredded carrots, broccoli florets, chopped baby bok choy, and cubed tofu. Cook for an additional 2•3 minutes until the vegetables are tender•crisp.

4. Divide the vegetable ramen between 4 bowls. Garnish with sliced green onions and toasted sesame seeds.

This vegetable ramen is a nutritious and flavorful meatless option that teens will enjoy. The miso paste, soy sauce, and sesame oil create a savory, umami•rich broth, while the variety of fresh vegetables add color, texture, and nutrients.

The cubed tofu provides plant•based protein to make this a filling and satisfying meal. The green onions and sesame seeds add a nice finishing touch. Feel free to swap in or add other vegetables based on your preferences, such as snow peas, bean sprouts, or spinach. You can also top it with a soft•boiled egg for extra protein.

23. Tofu Ramen

Ingredient:

• 6 cups vegetable broth
• 2 tablespoons soy sauce
• 1 tablespoon mirin
• 1 teaspoon sesame oil
• 1 garlic clove, minced
• 1•inch piece fresh ginger, peeled and grated
• 8 oz ramen noodles
• 1 block firm or extra•firm tofu, cubed
• 1 cup sliced mushrooms
• 1 cup shredded carrots
• 1 cup baby spinach or chopped kale
• Sliced green onions, for garnish
• Toasted sesame seeds, for garnish

Instructions:

1. In a large pot, combine the vegetable broth, soy sauce, mirin, sesame oil, garlic, and ginger. Bring to a simmer over medium heat.

2. Add the ramen noodles and cook according to package instructions, usually 2•3 minutes.

3. Stir in the cubed tofu, sliced mushrooms, shredded carrots, and baby spinach or kale. Cook for an additional 1•2 minutes until the greens are wilted.

4. Divide the tofu ramen between 4 bowls. Garnish with sliced green onions and toasted sesame seeds.

This tofu ramen is a delicious vegetarian option that's packed with protein and nutrients. The firm or extra•firm tofu provides a satisfying texture, while the vegetables add color, crunch, and vitamins.

The savory broth is seasoned with soy sauce, mirin, and aromatic garlic and ginger, giving it a rich, umami flavor. The green onions and sesame seeds add a fresh, nutty finishing touch.

Teens who are looking for a meatless ramen option or want to incorporate more plant•based proteins into their diet will enjoy this tofu ramen. Feel free to adjust the vegetables or add other toppings like soft•boiled eggs or crispy fried onions.

24. Quinoa Ramen

Ingredient:

- 6 cups chicken or vegetable broth
- 1 cup cooked quinoa
- 2 tablespoons low•sodium soy sauce
- 1 tablespoon rice vinegar
- 1 teaspoon sesame oil
- 1 garlic clove, minced
- 1•inch piece fresh ginger, peeled and grated
- 8 oz ramen noodles (or quinoa ramen noodles)
- 1 cup shredded cooked chicken or tofu
- 1 cup sliced mushrooms
- 1 cup shredded carrots
- 1 cup baby spinach or chopped kale
- Sliced green onions, for garnish
- Toasted sesame seeds, for garnish

Instructions:

1. In a large pot, combine the broth, cooked quinoa, soy sauce, rice vinegar, sesame oil, garlic, and ginger. Bring to a simmer over medium heat.

2. Add the ramen noodles and cook according to package instructions, usually 2•3 minutes.

3. Stir in the shredded chicken or tofu, sliced mushrooms, shredded carrots, and baby spinach or kale. Cook for an additional 1•2 minutes until the greens are wilted.

4. Divide the quinoa ramen between 4 bowls. Garnish with sliced green onions and toasted sesame seeds.

This quinoa ramen is a nutritious twist on the classic dish. The addition of cooked quinoa adds extra protein, fiber, and nutrients to the broth. You can use regular ramen noodles or opt for quinoa•based ramen noodles for an even healthier option.

The shredded chicken or tofu, mushrooms, carrots, and greens provide a variety of textures and flavors, making this a well•rounded and satisfying meal for teens.

The soy sauce, rice vinegar, and sesame oil give the broth a savory, umami•forward taste, while the green onions and sesame seeds add a fresh, crunchy garnish. Feel free to adjust the protein or vegetable toppings to your liking. This quinoa ramen is a great way to introduce teens to the benefits of this superfood grain.

25. Whole Wheat Ramen

Ingredient:

• 6 cups chicken or vegetable broth
• 2 tablespoons low•sodium soy sauce
• 1 tablespoon mirin
• 1 teaspoon sesame oil
• 1 garlic clove, minced
• 1•inch piece fresh ginger, peeled and grated
• 8 oz whole wheat ramen noodles
• 1 cup shredded cooked chicken or tofu
• 1 cup sliced mushrooms
• 1 cup shredded carrots
• 1 cup baby spinach or chopped kale
• Sliced green onions, for garnish
• Toasted sesame seeds, for garnish

Instructions:

1. In a large pot, combine the broth, soy sauce, mirin, sesame oil, garlic, and ginger. Bring to a simmer over medium heat.

2. Add the whole wheat ramen noodles and cook according to package instructions, usually 2•3 minutes.

3. Stir in the shredded chicken or tofu, sliced mushrooms, shredded carrots, and baby spinach or kale. Cook for an additional 1•2 minutes until the greens are wilted.

4. Divide the whole wheat ramen between 4 bowls. Garnish with sliced green onions and toasted sesame seeds.

This whole wheat ramen is a healthier twist on the classic dish. Whole wheat ramen noodles provide more fiber and nutrients compared to traditional white ramen.

The flavorful broth is seasoned with low•sodium soy sauce, mirin, and aromatic garlic and ginger. The shredded chicken or tofu, mushrooms, carrots, and greens add protein, vitamins, and minerals.

The green onions and sesame seeds provide a fresh, crunchy garnish. This ramen is a nutritious and satisfying meal that teens will enjoy. Feel free to adjust the protein or vegetable toppings to your liking. You can also add a soft•boiled egg or other garnishes to customize the dish.

26. Zoodle (Zucchini Noodle) Ramen

Ingredient:

• 6 cups chicken or vegetable broth
• 2 tablespoons low•sodium soy sauce
• 1 tablespoon rice vinegar
• 1 teaspoon sesame oil
• 1 garlic clove, minced
• 1•inch piece fresh ginger, peeled and grated
• 4 medium zucchinis, spiralized into noodles
• 1 cup shredded cooked chicken or tofu
• 1 cup sliced mushrooms
• 1 cup shredded carrots
• 1 cup baby spinach or chopped kale
• Sliced green onions, for garnish
• Toasted sesame seeds, for garnish

Instructions:

1. In a large pot, combine the broth, soy sauce, rice vinegar, sesame oil, garlic, and ginger. Bring to a simmer over medium heat.

2. Add the spiralized zucchini noodles and cook for 2•3 minutes, just until they start to soften.

3. Stir in the shredded chicken or tofu, sliced mushrooms, shredded carrots, and baby spinach or kale. Cook for an additional 1•2 minutes until the greens are wilted.

4. Divide the zoodle ramen between 4 bowls.

5. Garnish with sliced green onions and toasted sesame seeds.

This zoodle ramen is a low•carb, veggie•packed twist on traditional ramen. The spiralized zucchini noodles provide a healthier alternative to wheat•based ramen noodles, while still delivering the comforting texture and flavor.

The savory broth is seasoned with soy sauce, rice vinegar, and aromatic garlic and ginger. The shredded chicken or tofu, mushrooms, carrots, and greens add protein, fiber, and nutrients.

27. Kale Ramen

Ingredient:

- 6 cups chicken or vegetable broth
- 2 tablespoons miso paste
- 1 tablespoon soy sauce
- 1 teaspoon sesame oil
- 1 garlic clove, minced
- 1·inch piece fresh ginger, peeled and grated
- 8 oz ramen noodles
- 2 cups chopped kale
- 1 cup sliced mushrooms
- 1 cup shredded carrots
- 1 cup cubed firm tofu
- Sliced green onions, for garnish
- Toasted sesame seeds, for garnish

Instructions:

1. In a large pot, whisk together the broth, miso paste, soy sauce, sesame oil, garlic, and ginger. Bring to a simmer over medium heat.

2. Add the ramen noodles and cook according to package instructions, usually 2·3 minutes.

3. Stir in the chopped kale, sliced mushrooms, shredded carrots, and cubed tofu. Cook for an additional 2·3 minutes until the kale is wilted and the vegetables are tender.

4. Divide the kale ramen between 4 bowls. Garnish with sliced green onions and toasted sesame seeds.

This kale ramen is a nutrient·dense and flavorful option for teens. The miso paste, soy sauce, and sesame oil create a savory, umami·rich broth that complements the earthy kale.

The tofu provides plant·based protein, while the mushrooms, carrots, and kale add a variety of vitamins, minerals, and antioxidants. The green onions and sesame seeds add a fresh, crunchy garnish.

Kale is a superfood that's packed with nutrients like vitamin K, vitamin A, vitamin C, and calcium. Incorporating it into a comforting ramen dish is a great way to encourage teens to eat more greens.

28. Broccoli Ramen

Ingredient:

- 6 cups chicken or vegetable broth
- 2 tablespoons soy sauce
- 1 tablespoon rice vinegar
- 1 teaspoon sesame oil
- 1 garlic clove, minced
- 1-inch piece fresh ginger, peeled and grated
- 8 oz ramen noodles
- 2 cups broccoli florets
- 1 cup sliced mushrooms
- 1 cup shredded cooked chicken or tofu
- 2 green onions, sliced
- Sesame seeds, for garnish

Instructions:

1. In a large pot, combine the broth, soy sauce, rice vinegar, sesame oil, garlic, and ginger. Bring to a simmer over medium heat.

2. Add the ramen noodles and cook according to package instructions, usually 2-3 minutes.

3. Stir in the broccoli florets and sliced mushrooms. Cook for an additional 2-3 minutes until the broccoli is tender-crisp.

4. Remove from heat and stir in the shredded chicken or tofu.

5. Divide the broccoli ramen between 4 bowls.

6. Garnish with sliced green onions and sesame seeds.

This broccoli ramen is a nutritious and flavorful twist on classic ramen. The broccoli florets add a nice crunch and plenty of vitamins, while the mushrooms and protein-rich chicken or tofu make it a satisfying meal.

The broth is seasoned with soy sauce, rice vinegar, and aromatic garlic and ginger, giving it a savory, umami-forward flavor. The green onions and sesame seeds provide a fresh, nutty garnish.

29. Spinach Ramen

Ingredient:

• 2 packages of ramen noodles (discard the seasoning packets)
• 4 cups chicken or vegetable broth
• 2 cups fresh spinach, roughly chopped
• 2 eggs, soft•boiled or poached
• 2 green onions, sliced
• 1 tbsp soy sauce
• 1 tsp sesame oil
• 1 tsp rice vinegar
• 1 clove garlic, minced
• 1/2 tsp grated ginger
• Salt and pepper to taste
• Sesame seeds for garnish

Instructions:

1. In a large pot, bring the chicken or vegetable broth to a boil. Add the ramen noodles and cook for 2•3 minutes, until tender.

2. Stir in the chopped spinach and cook for an additional 1•2 minutes, until the spinach is wilted.

3. In a small bowl, whisk together the soy sauce, sesame oil, rice vinegar, minced garlic, and grated ginger.

4. Remove the pot from heat and stir in the soy sauce mixture until well combined.

5. Ladle the Spinach Ramen into bowls and top each serving with a soft•boiled or poached egg, sliced green onions, and a sprinkle of sesame seeds.

6. Season with salt and pepper to taste.

Enjoy your delicious and nutritious Spinach Ramen! This recipe is suitable for teens as it provides a healthy, vegetable•based option that is still flavorful and satisfying.

30. Cauliflower Ramen

Ingredient:

• 2 packages of ramen noodles (discard the seasoning packets)
• 1 head of cauliflower, cut into florets
• 4 cups vegetable or chicken broth
• 2 tbsp soy sauce
• 1 tbsp rice vinegar
• 1 tbsp honey
• 1 tsp sesame oil
• 2 cloves garlic, minced
• 1 inch piece of ginger, grated
• 2 green onions, sliced
• 1 soft•boiled egg (optional)
• Sesame seeds for garnish

Instructions:

1. In a large pot, bring the vegetable or chicken broth to a boil. Add the cauliflower florets and cook for 5•7 minutes, until the cauliflower is tender.

2. Using a slotted spoon, transfer the cooked cauliflower to a blender. Add 1 cup of the cooking broth, soy sauce, rice vinegar, honey, and sesame oil. Blend until smooth and creamy.

3. Return the blended cauliflower mixture to the pot with the remaining broth. Bring the mixture to a simmer.

4. Add the ramen noodles to the pot and cook for 2•3 minutes, until the noodles are tender.

5. Stir in the minced garlic and grated ginger. Cook for an additional 1•2 minutes.

6. Serve the Cauliflower Ramen in bowls, topped with sliced green onions, a soft•boiled egg (if using), and a sprinkle of sesame seeds.

Enjoy your delicious and nutritious Cauliflower Ramen! This recipe is suitable for teens as it provides a healthy, vegetable•based alternative to traditional ramen.

31. Mexican Ramen

Ingredient:

• 2 packages of ramen noodles (discard the seasoning packets)
• 1 lb ground beef or turkey
• 1 onion, diced
• 2 cloves garlic, minced
• 1 tbsp chili powder
• 1 tsp cumin
• 1 tsp oregano
• 1/2 tsp smoked paprika
• 1/4 tsp cayenne pepper (optional, for a bit of heat)
• 4 cups chicken or vegetable broth
• 1 cup diced tomatoes (canned or fresh)
• 1 cup shredded cheddar or Monterey Jack cheese
• 2 green onions, sliced
• Chopped cilantro for garnish
• Lime wedges for serving

Instructions:

1. In a large pot or skillet, cook the ground beef or turkey over medium•high heat, breaking it up as it cooks, until browned and cooked through, about 5•7 minutes.

2. Add the diced onion and minced garlic to the pot and cook for 2•3 minutes, until the onion is translucent.

3. Stir in the chili powder, cumin, oregano, smoked paprika, and cayenne pepper (if using). Cook for 1 minute to toast the spices.

4. Pour in the chicken or vegetable broth and diced tomatoes. Bring the mixture to a simmer.

5. Add the ramen noodles to the pot and cook for 2•3 minutes, until the noodles are tender.

6. Remove the pot from heat and stir in the shredded cheese until it's melted and well combined.

7. Serve the Mexican Ramen in bowls, topped with sliced green onions and chopped cilantro. Serve with lime wedges on the side.

32. Italian Ramen

Ingredient:

- 2 packages of ramen noodles (discard the seasoning packets)
- 1 lb ground Italian sausage, casings removed
- 2 cloves garlic, minced
- 1 onion, diced
- 1 cup diced tomatoes (canned or fresh)
- 2 cups chicken or vegetable broth
- 1 tsp dried oregano
- 1 tsp dried basil
- 1/2 tsp red pepper flakes (optional, for a bit of heat)
- 1 cup shredded mozzarella cheese
- 2 tbsp grated Parmesan cheese
- Fresh basil leaves for garnish

Instructions:

1. In a large pot or skillet, cook the ground Italian sausage over medium•high heat, breaking it up as it cooks, until browned and cooked through, about 5•7 minutes.

2. Add the minced garlic and diced onion to the pot and cook for 2•3 minutes, until the onion is translucent.

3. Stir in the diced tomatoes, chicken or vegetable broth, dried oregano, dried basil, and red pepper flakes (if using). Bring the mixture to a simmer.

4. Add the ramen noodles to the pot and cook for 2•3 minutes, until the noodles are tender.

5. Remove the pot from heat and stir in the shredded mozzarella cheese until it's melted and well combined.

6. Serve the Italian Ramen in bowls, topped with grated Parmesan cheese and fresh basil leaves.

Enjoy your delicious and comforting Italian•inspired Ramen! This recipe is suitable for teens as it has a mild, savory, and slightly spicy flavor profile.

33. Indian Curry Ramen

Ingredient:

• 2 packages of ramen noodles (discard the seasoning packets)
• 1 tbsp vegetable oil
• 1 onion, diced
• 2 cloves garlic, minced
• 1 tbsp grated ginger
• 2 tsp curry powder
• 1 tsp garam masala
• 1/2 tsp turmeric
• 1/4 tsp cayenne pepper (optional, for a bit of heat)
• 4 cups chicken or vegetable broth
• 1 cup canned diced tomatoes
• 1 cup cooked chickpeas (or other protein of your choice)
• 1 cup frozen peas
• 2 tbsp chopped cilantro
• Lime wedges for serving

Instructions:

1. In a large pot or skillet, heat the vegetable oil over medium heat. Add the diced onion and cook for 3•4 minutes, until translucent.

2. Add the minced garlic and grated ginger to the pot and cook for 1 minute, until fragrant.

3. Stir in the curry powder, garam masala, turmeric, and cayenne pepper (if using). Cook for 1 minute to toast the spices.

4. Pour in the chicken or vegetable broth and the diced tomatoes. Bring the mixture to a simmer.

5. Add the ramen noodles and cook for 2•3 minutes, until the noodles are tender.

6. Stir in the cooked chickpeas (or other protein) and frozen peas. Cook for an additional 2•3 minutes, until the peas are heated through.

7. Remove the pot from heat and stir in the chopped cilantro. Serve the Indian Curry Ramen in bowls, with lime wedges on the side.

Enjoy your delicious and flavorful Indian•inspired Ramen! This recipe is suitable for teens as it has a moderate level of spice that can be adjusted to their preference.

34. Korean BBQ Ramen

Ingredient:

• 2 packages of ramen noodles (discard the seasoning packets)
• 1 lb boneless, skinless chicken thighs, thinly sliced
• 2 tbsp gochujang (Korean red chili paste)
• 2 tbsp soy sauce
• 1 tbsp brown sugar
• 1 tbsp sesame oil
• 2 cloves garlic, minced
• 1 inch piece of ginger, grated
• 4 cups chicken or vegetable broth
• 2 cups shredded cabbage
• 2 green onions, sliced
• 1 soft•boiled egg (optional)
• Sesame seeds for garnish

Instructions:

1. In a bowl, combine the sliced chicken, gochujang, soy sauce, brown sugar, sesame oil, garlic, and ginger. Mix well and let marinate for 15•20 minutes.

2. In a large pot, bring the broth to a boil. Add the ramen noodles and cook for 2•3 minutes until tender.

3. Add the marinated chicken and cook for 5•7 minutes, until the chicken is cooked through.

4. Stir in the shredded cabbage and green onions. Cook for an additional 2•3 minutes.

5. Serve the Korean BBQ ramen in bowls, topped with a soft•boiled egg (if using) and a sprinkle of sesame seeds.

Enjoy your delicious and flavorful Korean BBQ Ramen! This recipe is suitable for teens as it has a moderate level of spice from the gochujang.

35. Mediterranean Ramen

Ingredient:

• 2 packages of ramen noodles (discard the seasoning packets)
• 4 cups chicken or vegetable broth
• 1 cup diced tomatoes (canned or fresh)
• 1 cup cooked chickpeas
• 1/2 cup crumbled feta cheese
• 1/4 cup kalamata olives, sliced
• 2 tbsp chopped fresh parsley
• 1 tbsp lemon juice
• 1 tsp dried oregano
• 1 tsp olive oil
• 1 clove garlic, minced
• Salt and pepper to taste

Instructions:

1. In a large pot, bring the chicken or vegetable broth to a boil. Add the ramen noodles and cook for 2•3 minutes, until tender.

2. Drain the ramen noodles and return them to the pot.

3. Add the diced tomatoes, cooked chickpeas, crumbled feta cheese, sliced kalamata olives, chopped parsley, lemon juice, dried oregano, olive oil, and minced garlic to the pot. Stir to combine.

4. Season with salt and pepper to taste.

5. Serve the Mediterranean Ramen warm, garnished with additional parsley or feta cheese if desired.

Enjoy your delicious and flavorful Mediterranean•inspired Ramen! This recipe is suitable for teens as it has a fresh, tangy, and slightly salty flavor profile that is often enjoyed by young adults.

36. Teriyaki Ramen

Ingredient:

• 2 packages of ramen noodles (discard the seasoning packets)
• 1 lb boneless, skinless chicken thighs, cut into bite•sized pieces
• 2 tbsp teriyaki sauce
• 1 tbsp brown sugar
• 1 tbsp soy sauce
• 1 tsp sesame oil
• 2 cloves garlic, minced
• 1 inch piece of ginger, grated
• 4 cups chicken or vegetable broth
• 2 cups shredded cabbage
• 2 green onions, sliced
• 1 soft•boiled egg (optional)
• Sesame seeds for garnish

Instructions:

1. In a bowl, combine the diced chicken, teriyaki sauce, brown sugar, soy sauce, sesame oil, garlic, and ginger. Mix well and let marinate for 15•20 minutes.

2. In a large pot, bring the broth to a boil. Add the ramen noodles and cook for 2•3 minutes until tender.

3. Add the marinated chicken and cook for 5•7 minutes, until the chicken is cooked through.

4. Stir in the shredded cabbage and green onions. Cook for an additional 2•3 minutes.

5. Serve the Teriyaki Ramen in bowls, topped with a soft•boiled egg (if using) and a sprinkle of sesame seeds.

Enjoy your delicious and flavorful Teriyaki Ramen! This recipe is suitable for teens as it has a mild, sweet, and savory flavor profile.

37. Pesto Ramen

Ingredient:

• 2 packages of ramen noodles (discard the seasoning packets)
• 4 cups chicken or vegetable broth
• 1/2 cup prepared basil pesto
• 1 cup cherry tomatoes, halved
• 1 cup shredded rotisserie chicken (or cooked chicken of your choice)
• 1/2 cup shredded mozzarella cheese
• 2 tbsp toasted pine nuts
• 2 tbsp grated Parmesan cheese
• 2 tbsp chopped fresh basil
• Salt and pepper to taste

Instructions:

1. In a large pot, bring the chicken or vegetable broth to a boil. Add the ramen noodles and cook for 2•3 minutes, until tender.

2. Drain the ramen noodles and return them to the pot.

3. Add the prepared basil pesto to the pot and stir to coat the noodles evenly.

4. Stir in the halved cherry tomatoes, shredded rotisserie chicken, shredded mozzarella cheese, toasted pine nuts, and grated Parmesan cheese.

5. Cook for an additional 1•2 minutes, just until the cheese starts to melt.

6. Remove the pot from heat and stir in the chopped fresh basil.

7. Season with salt and pepper to taste.

8. Serve the Pesto Ramen warm, garnished with additional basil if desired.

Enjoy your delicious and flavorful Pesto Ramen! This recipe is suitable for teens as it combines the familiar comfort of ramen with the fresh, herbal flavors of pesto.

38. Taco Ramen

Ingredient:

- 2 packages of ramen noodles (discard the seasoning packets)
- 1 lb ground beef or turkey
- 1 packet taco seasoning
- 4 cups chicken or beef broth
- 1 cup diced tomatoes (canned or fresh)
- 1 cup shredded lettuce
- 1/2 cup shredded cheddar or Monterey Jack cheese
- 2 tbsp chopped cilantro
- 1 avocado, diced
- Crushed tortilla chips for garnish
- Lime wedges for serving

Instructions:

1. In a large skillet, cook the ground beef or turkey over medium-high heat, breaking it up as it cooks, until browned and cooked through, about 5-7 minutes.

2. Drain any excess fat from the skillet, then add the taco seasoning and stir to coat the meat.

3. In a large pot, bring the chicken or beef broth to a boil. Add the ramen noodles and cook for 2-3 minutes, until tender.

4. Stir the cooked taco meat into the pot with the ramen noodles. Add the diced tomatoes and let the mixture simmer for 2-3 minutes.

5. Remove the pot from heat and stir in the shredded lettuce, shredded cheese, and chopped cilantro.

6. Serve the Taco Ramen in bowls, topped with diced avocado and crushed tortilla chips. Serve with lime wedges on the side.

Enjoy your delicious and flavorful Taco Ramen! This recipe is suitable for teens as it combines the familiar flavors of tacos with the comfort of ramen noodles.

39. Pizza Ramen

Ingredient:

- 2 packages of ramen noodles (discard the seasoning packets)
- 4 cups chicken or vegetable broth
- 1 cup marinara sauce
- 1/2 cup diced pepperoni
- 1/2 cup sliced mushrooms
- 1/2 cup diced bell pepper
- 1/2 cup shredded mozzarella cheese
- 2 tbsp grated Parmesan cheese
- 2 tbsp chopped fresh basil
- Salt and pepper to taste

Instructions:

1. In a large pot, bring the chicken or vegetable broth to a boil. Add the ramen noodles and cook for 2•3 minutes, until tender.

2. Drain the ramen noodles and return them to the pot.

3. Stir in the marinara sauce, diced pepperoni, sliced mushrooms, and diced bell pepper. Heat the mixture over medium heat for 2•3 minutes, until the vegetables are slightly softened.

4. Remove the pot from heat and stir in the shredded mozzarella cheese and grated Parmesan cheese until melted and well combined.

5. Serve the Pizza Ramen warm, garnished with chopped fresh basil.

6. Season with salt and pepper to taste.

Enjoy your delicious and satisfying Pizza Ramen! This recipe is suitable for teens as it combines the familiar flavors of pizza with the comfort of ramen noodles.

40. Pad Thai Ramen

Ingredient:

- 6 cups chicken or vegetable broth
- 2 tablespoons tamarind paste
- 2 tablespoons fish sauce
- 1 tablespoon brown sugar
- 1 teaspoon chili•garlic sauce (or sriracha)
- 8 oz ramen noodles
- 1 cup cooked shrimp or tofu
- 1 cup bean sprouts
- 1 cup shredded carrots
- 1/2 cup chopped roasted peanuts
- 2 green onions, sliced
- 1/4 cup chopped cilantro
- Lime wedges, for serving

Instructions:

1. In a large pot, whisk together the broth, tamarind paste, fish sauce, brown sugar, and chili•garlic sauce. Bring to a simmer over medium heat.

2. Add the ramen noodles and cook according to package instructions, usually 2•3 minutes.

3. Stir in the cooked shrimp or tofu, bean sprouts, and shredded carrots. Cook for an additional 1•2 minutes until heated through.

4. Divide the pad thai ramen between 4 bowls.

5. Top each bowl with chopped roasted peanuts, sliced green onions, and chopped cilantro.

6. Serve with lime wedges on the side.

This pad thai ramen combines the flavors of classic pad thai with the comforting noodles and broth of ramen. The tamarind paste, fish sauce, and brown sugar create a sweet, sour, and savory sauce that coats the noodles.

The shrimp or tofu, bean sprouts, and carrots add protein, crunch, and freshness. The roasted peanuts, green onions, and cilantro provide a flavorful garnish.

41. Instant Ramen Upgrade

Ingredient:

• 1 package of instant ramen noodles (discard the seasoning packet)
• 1 cup boiling water
• 1 egg
• 1/2 cup frozen mixed vegetables (such as peas, carrots, and corn)
• 2 tbsp chopped cooked chicken or tofu (optional)
• 1 tbsp soy sauce
• 1 tsp sesame oil
• 1 tsp sriracha or other hot sauce (optional)
• Chopped green onions for garnish

Instructions:

1. In a large microwave•safe mug or bowl, place the instant ramen noodles.

2. Pour the boiling water over the noodles and let them sit for 2•3 minutes, until the noodles are tender.

3. Crack the egg into the mug or bowl with the noodles and stir gently to partially cook the egg.

4. Add the frozen mixed vegetables, cooked chicken or tofu (if using), soy sauce, sesame oil, and sriracha (if using) to the mug or bowl. Stir to combine.

5. Microwave the ramen for an additional 1•2 minutes, or until the egg is fully cooked and the vegetables are heated through.

6. Carefully remove the mug or bowl from the microwave and stir the ramen one more time.

7. Serve the Instant Ramen Upgrade immediately, garnished with chopped green onions.

Enjoy your upgraded instant ramen! This recipe is suitable for teens as it's a quick and easy way to add some extra flavor and nutrition to a basic instant ramen dish.

42. Microwave Ramen

Ingredient:

- 1 package of ramen noodles (discard the seasoning packet)
- 1 cup water
- 1 egg
- 1/2 cup frozen mixed vegetables (such as peas, carrots, and corn)
- 1 tbsp soy sauce
- 1 tsp sesame oil
- 1 tsp sriracha or other hot sauce (optional)
- Chopped green onions for garnish

Instructions:

1. In a microwave·safe bowl, combine the ramen noodles and 1 cup of water.

2. Microwave the noodles for 2·3 minutes, or until the noodles are tender.

3. Carefully remove the bowl from the microwave (it will be hot!) and crack the egg into the bowl with the noodles. Stir the egg into the hot noodles until it's partially cooked.

4. Add the frozen mixed vegetables, soy sauce, sesame oil, and sriracha (if using) to the bowl. Stir to combine.

5. Microwave the ramen for an additional 1·2 minutes, or until the vegetables are heated through and the egg is fully cooked.

6. Carefully remove the bowl from the microwave and stir the ramen one more time.

7. Serve the Microwave Ramen immediately, garnished with chopped green onions.

Enjoy your quick and easy Microwave Ramen! This recipe is suitable for teens as it's a simple, customizable, and convenient option for a quick meal.

43. One•Pot Ramen

Ingredient:

• 2 packages of ramen noodles (discard the seasoning packets)
• 4 cups chicken or vegetable broth
• 1 lb boneless, skinless chicken thighs, cut into bite•sized pieces
• 2 cups sliced mushrooms
• 1 cup shredded cabbage
• 2 green onions, sliced
• 2 tbsp soy sauce
• 1 tbsp rice vinegar
• 1 tsp sesame oil
• 1 tsp grated ginger
• 2 cloves garlic, minced
• Salt and pepper to taste
• Soft•boiled eggs (optional)
• Sesame seeds for garnish

Instructions:

1. In a large pot, combine the chicken or vegetable broth, chicken pieces, sliced mushrooms, shredded cabbage, green onions, soy sauce, rice vinegar, sesame oil, grated ginger, and minced garlic.

2. Bring the mixture to a boil over high heat, then reduce the heat to medium•low and let it simmer for 10•12 minutes, or until the chicken is cooked through and the vegetables are tender.

3. Add the ramen noodles to the pot and cook for an additional 2•3 minutes, until the noodles are tender.

4. Remove the pot from heat and season with salt and pepper to taste.

5. Serve the One•Pot Ramen warm, topped with soft•boiled eggs (if using) and a sprinkle of sesame seeds.

Enjoy your delicious and easy•to•make One•Pot Ramen! This recipe is suitable for teens as it's a complete, one•dish meal that's both comforting and flavorful.

44. Stir•Fry Ramen

Ingredient:

• 2 packages of ramen noodles (discard the seasoning packets)
• 2 tbsp vegetable oil
• 1 lb boneless, skinless chicken thighs, cut into bite•sized pieces
• 2 cloves garlic, minced
• 1 inch piece of ginger, grated
• 1 cup sliced mushrooms
• 1 cup sliced bell peppers
• 1 cup shredded cabbage
• 2 tbsp soy sauce
• 1 tbsp rice vinegar
• 1 tsp sesame oil
• 2 green onions, sliced
• Sesame seeds for garnish

Instructions:

1. Bring a large pot of water to a boil. Add the ramen noodles and cook according to package instructions, about 2•3 minutes. Drain and set aside.

2. In a large skillet or wok, heat the vegetable oil over high heat. Add the chicken and cook for 3•4 minutes, until lightly browned.

3. Add the minced garlic and grated ginger to the skillet and cook for 1 minute, until fragrant.

4. Stir in the sliced mushrooms, bell peppers, and shredded cabbage. Cook for 3•4 minutes, until the vegetables are tender•crisp.

5. Add the cooked ramen noodles, soy sauce, rice vinegar, and sesame oil to the skillet. Toss everything together until well combined and heated through.

6. Remove from heat and stir in the sliced green onions.

7. Serve the Stir•Fry Ramen immediately, garnished with sesame seeds.

Enjoy your delicious and flavorful Stir•Fry Ramen! This recipe is suitable for teens as it provides a healthy, veggie•packed option that is still satisfying and easy to prepare.

45. Mug Ramen

Ingredient:

• 1 package of instant ramen noodles (discard the seasoning packet)
• 1 cup boiling water
• 1 egg
• 1/2 cup frozen mixed vegetables (such as peas, carrots, and corn)
• 2 tbsp cooked chicken or tofu, chopped (optional)
• 1 tbsp soy sauce
• 1 tsp sesame oil
• 1 tsp sriracha or other hot sauce (optional)
• Chopped green onions for garnish

Instructions:

1. In a large microwave•safe mug or bowl, place the instant ramen noodles.

2. Pour the boiling water over the noodles and let them sit for 2•3 minutes, until the noodles are tender.

3. Crack the egg into the mug or bowl with the noodles and stir gently to partially cook the egg.

4. Add the frozen mixed vegetables, cooked chicken or tofu (if using), soy sauce, sesame oil, and sriracha (if using) to the mug or bowl. Stir to combine.

5. Microwave the ramen for an additional 1•2 minutes, or until the egg is fully cooked and the vegetables are heated through.

6. Carefully remove the mug or bowl from the microwave and stir the ramen one more time.

7. Serve the Mug Ramen immediately, garnished with chopped green onions.

Enjoy your quick and easy Mug Ramen! This recipe is suitable for teens as it's a simple, customizable, and convenient option for a quick meal.

46. Ramen Salad

Ingredient:

• 2 packages of ramen noodles, crushed (discard the seasoning packets)
• 1 cup shredded cabbage
• 1 cup shredded carrots
• 1/2 cup sliced green onions
• 1/4 cup toasted slivered almonds
• 2 tbsp sesame seeds
• 2 tbsp vegetable oil
• 2 tbsp rice vinegar
• 1 tbsp soy sauce
• 1 tsp sesame oil
• 1 tsp honey
• Salt and pepper to taste

Instructions:

1. In a large bowl, combine the crushed ramen noodles, shredded cabbage, shredded carrots, sliced green onions, toasted slivered almonds, and sesame seeds.

2. In a small bowl, whisk together the vegetable oil, rice vinegar, soy sauce, sesame oil, and honey.

3. Pour the dressing over the ramen salad and toss to coat everything evenly.

4. Season the salad with salt and pepper to taste.

5. Cover the bowl and refrigerate the Ramen Salad for at least 30 minutes to allow the flavors to meld.

6. Serve the chilled Ramen Salad as a side dish or a light main course.

Enjoy your refreshing and crunchy Ramen Salad! This recipe is suitable for teens as it provides a healthy, flavorful alternative to traditional ramen dishes.

47. Cold Ramen Noodles

Ingredient:

• 2 packages of ramen noodles (discard the seasoning packets)
• 2 cups shredded cooked chicken or tofu (optional)
• 1 cup shredded cabbage
• 1 cup shredded carrots
• 1/2 cup sliced cucumber
• 2 green onions, sliced
• 2 tbsp sesame seeds
• 2 tbsp soy sauce
• 2 tbsp rice vinegar
• 1 tbsp sesame oil
• 1 tsp honey
• Salt and pepper to taste

Instructions:

1. Bring a large pot of water to a boil. Add the ramen noodles and cook according to package instructions, about 2•3 minutes. Drain the noodles and rinse them under cold water until they are completely cooled.

2. In a large bowl, combine the cooked and cooled ramen noodles, shredded chicken or tofu (if using), shredded cabbage, shredded carrots, sliced cucumber, and sliced green onions.

3. In a small bowl, whisk together the sesame seeds, soy sauce, rice vinegar, sesame oil, and honey.

4. Pour the dressing over the ramen noodle mixture and toss to coat everything evenly.

5. Season the Cold Ramen Noodles with salt and pepper to taste.

6. Cover the bowl and refrigerate the noodles for at least 30 minutes to allow the flavors to meld.

7. Serve the chilled Cold Ramen Noodles as a refreshing main dish or side.

Enjoy your delicious and flavorful Cold Ramen Noodles! This recipe is suitable for teens as it provides a light and healthy option for a hot summer day.

48. Ramen Omelette

Ingredient:

- 1 package of ramen noodles (discard the seasoning packet)
- 3 eggs
- 2 tbsp milk
- 1 tbsp butter
- 2 tbsp shredded cheese (cheddar, mozzarella, or a blend)
- 2 tbsp chopped green onions
- Salt and pepper to taste

Instructions:

1. Bring a small pot of water to a boil. Add the ramen noodles and cook for 2•3 minutes, until tender. Drain the noodles and set aside.

2. In a small bowl, whisk together the eggs and milk. Season with a pinch of salt and pepper.

3. In a nonstick skillet, melt the butter over medium heat.

4. Pour the egg mixture into the skillet and let it cook for 1•2 minutes, until the edges start to set.

5. Sprinkle the cooked ramen noodles, shredded cheese, and chopped green onions over the top of the egg mixture.

6. Use a spatula to gently fold the omelette in half, then slide it onto a plate.

7. Serve the Ramen Omelette warm, garnished with additional green onions if desired.

Enjoy your creative and delicious Ramen Omelette! This recipe is suitable for teens as it combines the comfort of ramen noodles with the classic breakfast dish of an omelette.

49. Ramen Stir•Fry

Ingredient:

• 2 packages of ramen noodles (discard the seasoning packets)
• 2 tbsp vegetable oil
• 1 lb boneless, skinless chicken thighs, cut into bite•sized pieces
• 2 cloves garlic, minced
• 1 inch piece of ginger, grated
• 1 cup sliced mushrooms
• 1 cup sliced bell peppers
• 1 cup shredded cabbage
• 2 tbsp soy sauce
• 1 tbsp rice vinegar
• 1 tsp sesame oil
• 2 green onions, sliced
• Sesame seeds for garnish

Instructions:

1. Bring a large pot of water to a boil. Add the ramen noodles and cook according to package instructions, about 2•3 minutes. Drain and set aside.

2. In a large skillet or wok, heat the vegetable oil over high heat. Add the chicken and cook for 3•4 minutes, until lightly browned.

3. Add the minced garlic and grated ginger to the skillet and cook for 1 minute, until fragrant.

4. Stir in the sliced mushrooms, bell peppers, and shredded cabbage. Cook for 3•4 minutes, until the vegetables are tender•crisp.

5. Add the cooked ramen noodles, soy sauce, rice vinegar, and sesame oil to the skillet. Toss everything together until well combined and heated through.

6. Remove from heat and stir in the sliced green onions. Serve the Ramen Stir•Fry immediately, garnished with sesame seeds.

Enjoy your delicious and flavorful Ramen Stir•Fry! This recipe is suitable for teens as it provides a healthy, veggie•packed option that is still satisfying and easy to prepare.

50. Ramen Noodle Soup

Ingredient:

• 2 packages of ramen noodles (discard the seasoning packets)
• 4 cups chicken or vegetable broth
• 2 tbsp soy sauce
• 1 tbsp mirin (or rice vinegar)
• 1 tsp sesame oil
• 2 cloves garlic, minced
• 1 inch piece of ginger, grated
• 1 cup sliced mushrooms (such as shiitake or cremini)
• 1 cup shredded cooked chicken or tofu (optional)
• 2 cups baby spinach or bok choy
• 2 soft·boiled eggs (optional)
• Chopped green onions for garnish
• Sesame seeds for garnish

Instructions:

1. In a large pot, bring the chicken or vegetable broth to a boil. Add the ramen noodles and cook for 2·3 minutes, until tender.

2. Reduce the heat to low and stir in the soy sauce, mirin, sesame oil, minced garlic, and grated ginger. Simmer for 2·3 minutes to allow the flavors to meld.

3. Add the sliced mushrooms and shredded chicken or tofu (if using) to the pot. Cook for an additional 2·3 minutes, until the mushrooms are tender.

4. Stir in the baby spinach or bok choy and cook for 1 minute, just until the greens are wilted.

5. Serve the Ramen Noodle Soup warm, topped with a soft·boiled egg (if using), chopped green onions, and a sprinkle of sesame seeds.

Enjoy your comforting and flavorful Ramen Noodle Soup! This recipe is suitable for teens as it provides a simple, yet satisfying, ramen·based dish.

51. Truffle Ramen

Ingredient:

• 2 packages of ramen noodles (discard the seasoning packets)
• 4 cups chicken or vegetable broth
• 2 tbsp soy sauce
• 1 tbsp mirin (or rice vinegar)
• 1 tsp sesame oil
• 1 tsp truffle oil
• 2 cloves garlic, minced
• 1 inch piece of ginger, grated
• 4 oz shiitake mushrooms, sliced
• 2 cups baby spinach
• 2 soft•boiled eggs (optional)
• Chopped green onions for garnish
• Shaved truffle or truffle zest for garnish (optional)

Instructions:

1. In a large pot, bring the chicken or vegetable broth to a boil. Add the ramen noodles and cook for 2•3 minutes, until tender.

2. Drain the ramen noodles and return them to the pot.

3. Add the soy sauce, mirin, sesame oil, truffle oil, minced garlic, and grated ginger to the pot. Stir to combine.

4. Stir in the sliced shiitake mushrooms and baby spinach. Cook for an additional 1•2 minutes, until the spinach is wilted.

5. Serve the Truffle Ramen in bowls, topped with a soft•boiled egg (if using), chopped green onions, and shaved truffle or truffle zest (if using).

Enjoy your luxurious and flavorful Truffle Ramen! This recipe is suitable for teens as it provides a sophisticated twist on classic ramen, with the earthy and aromatic notes of truffle.

52. Lobster Ramen

Ingredient:

- 4 cups chicken or vegetable broth
- 2 tablespoons soy sauce
- 1 tablespoon mirin or rice vinegar
- 1 teaspoon sesame oil
- 1 teaspoon grated ginger
- 2 garlic cloves, minced
- 8 oz ramen noodles
- 8 oz cooked lobster meat, chopped
- 2 soft•boiled eggs, halved
- 2 green onions, sliced
- Sesame seeds for garnish

Instructions:

1. In a large pot, bring the broth, soy sauce, mirin, sesame oil, ginger, and garlic to a simmer over medium heat.

2. Add the ramen noodles and cook for 2•3 minutes until tender.

3. Remove from heat and stir in the chopped lobster meat.

4. Ladle the ramen into bowls and top each serving with a soft•boiled egg, sliced green onions, and a sprinkle of sesame seeds.

5. Serve hot and enjoy!

The rich, savory broth paired with the tender lobster meat makes this ramen dish feel extra luxurious. The soft•boiled egg and crunchy garnishes add great texture and flavor contrasts. This is a delicious way to enjoy ramen with a seafood twist.

53. Duck Ramen

Ingredient:

- 4 cups chicken or duck broth
- 2 tablespoons soy sauce
- 1 tablespoon mirin or rice vinegar
- 1 teaspoon sesame oil
- 2 garlic cloves, minced
- 1 inch ginger, grated
- 8 oz ramen noodles
- 8 oz roasted duck, shredded
- 2 soft•boiled eggs, halved
- 2 green onions, sliced
- Sesame seeds for garnish

Instructions:

1. In a large pot, bring the broth, soy sauce, mirin, sesame oil, garlic, and ginger to a simmer over medium heat.

2. Add the ramen noodles and cook for 2•3 minutes until tender.

3. Remove from heat and stir in the shredded roasted duck.

4. Ladle the ramen into bowls and top each serving with a soft•boiled egg, sliced green onions, and a sprinkle of sesame seeds.

5. Serve hot and enjoy!

The rich, savory duck broth paired with the tender shredded duck meat makes this ramen dish extra flavorful. The soft•boiled egg and crunchy garnishes add great texture and flavor contrasts. This is a delicious way to enjoy ramen with a poultry twist.

You can use either chicken or duck broth as the base, depending on your preference. Roasted duck legs or breasts work well for the shredded duck meat. This recipe makes for a hearty and satisfying ramen bowl.

54. Foie Gras Ramen

Ingredient:

• 4 cups chicken broth
• 2 tablespoons soy sauce
• 1 tablespoon mirin or rice vinegar
• 1 teaspoon sesame oil
• 2 garlic cloves, minced
• 1 inch ginger, grated
• 8 oz ramen noodles
• 2 cups shredded cooked chicken
• 2 soft•boiled eggs, halved
• 2 green onions, sliced
• Sesame seeds for garnish

Instructions:

1. In a large pot, bring the chicken broth, soy sauce, mirin, sesame oil, garlic, and ginger to a simmer over medium heat.

2. Add the ramen noodles and cook for 2•3 minutes until tender.

3. Remove from heat and stir in the shredded chicken.

4. Ladle the ramen into bowls and top each serving with a soft•boiled egg, sliced green onions, and a sprinkle of sesame seeds.

5. Serve hot and enjoy!

This chicken ramen recipe uses more accessible and family•friendly ingredients while still providing a delicious and satisfying ramen experience. Please let me know if you would like me to suggest any other teen•friendly ramen recipes.

55. Black Garlic Ramen

Ingredient:

• 2 packages of ramen noodles (discard the seasoning packets)
• 4 cups chicken or vegetable broth
• 4 cloves black garlic, minced (or 2 cloves regular garlic, minced)
• 2 tbsp soy sauce
• 1 tbsp mirin (or rice vinegar)
• 1 tsp sesame oil
• 1/2 tsp ground black pepper
• 1 cup shredded cooked chicken (or tofu for a vegetarian option)
• 2 cups baby spinach
• 2 soft•boiled eggs (optional)
• Sliced green onions for garnish
• Sesame seeds for garnish

Instructions:

1. In a large pot, bring the chicken or vegetable broth to a boil. Add the ramen noodles and cook for 2•3 minutes, until tender.

2. Drain the ramen noodles and return them to the pot.

3. Add the minced black garlic, soy sauce, mirin, sesame oil, and ground black pepper to the pot. Stir to combine.

4. Stir in the shredded cooked chicken (or tofu) and baby spinach. Cook for an additional 1•2 minutes, until the spinach is wilted.

5. Serve the Black Garlic Ramen in bowls, topped with a soft•boiled egg (if using), sliced green onions, and a sprinkle of sesame seeds.

Enjoy your delicious and flavorful Black Garlic Ramen! This recipe is suitable for teens as the black garlic provides a unique, savory•sweet flavor that is often enjoyed by young adults.

56. Wagyu Beef Ramen

Ingredient:

• 4 cups beef or chicken broth
• 2 tablespoons soy sauce
• 1 tablespoon mirin or rice vinegar
• 1 teaspoon sesame oil
• 2 garlic cloves, minced
• 1 inch ginger, grated
• 8 oz ramen noodles
• 8 oz thinly sliced wagyu beef
• 2 soft•boiled eggs, halved
• 2 green onions, sliced
• Sesame seeds for garnish

Instructions:

1. In a large pot, bring the broth, soy sauce, mirin, sesame oil, garlic, and ginger to a simmer over medium heat.

2. Add the ramen noodles and cook for 2•3 minutes until tender.

3. Remove from heat and gently stir in the thinly sliced wagyu beef. The residual heat will cook the beef.

4. Ladle the ramen into bowls and top each serving with a soft•boiled egg, sliced green onions, and a sprinkle of sesame seeds.

5. Serve hot and enjoy!

The rich, beefy broth paired with the tender, marbled wagyu beef makes this ramen dish extra luxurious. The soft•boiled egg and crunchy garnishes add great texture and flavor contrasts. This is a truly decadent way to enjoy ramen.

Wagyu beef is an extremely high•quality, well•marbled Japanese beef that has a melt•in•your•mouth texture. It can be quite expensive, so you can substitute with another high•quality beef if needed. The key is to slice it very thinly so it cooks quickly in the hot broth.

This recipe makes for an indulgent and satisfying ramen bowl that's sure to impress. Enjoy!

57. Sea Urchin Ramen

Ingredient:

• 4 cups seafood or chicken broth
• 2 tablespoons soy sauce
• 1 tablespoon mirin or rice vinegar
• 1 teaspoon sesame oil
• 2 garlic cloves, minced
• 1 inch ginger, grated
• 8 oz ramen noodles
• 4 oz fresh sea urchin (uni)
• 2 soft•boiled eggs, halved
• 2 green onions, sliced
• Sesame seeds for garnish

Instructions:

1. In a large pot, bring the broth, soy sauce, mirin, sesame oil, garlic, and ginger to a simmer over medium heat.

2. Add the ramen noodles and cook for 2•3 minutes until tender.

3. Remove from heat and gently fold in the fresh sea urchin. The residual heat will lightly cook the uni.

4. Ladle the ramen into bowls and top each serving with a soft•boiled egg, sliced green onions, and a sprinkle of sesame seeds.

5. Serve hot and enjoy!

The briny, creamy sea urchin adds a unique and delicate flavor to the savory ramen broth. The soft•boiled egg and crunchy garnishes provide great textural contrast. This dish is a bit more elevated than a typical teen ramen, but the ingredients are still accessible and appropriate.

Sea urchin can be found at some specialty seafood markets or Asian grocery stores. If it's not available, you can substitute with other types of seafood like shrimp, scallops, or even crab meat. Just be sure to adjust the cooking time accordingly.

58. Caviar Ramen

Ingredient:

- 4 cups vegetable or chicken broth
- 2 tablespoons white or yellow miso paste
- 1 tablespoon soy sauce
- 1 teaspoon sesame oil
- 2 garlic cloves, minced
- 1 inch ginger, grated
- 8 oz ramen noodles
- 1 cup sliced mushrooms
- 1 cup shredded cooked chicken or tofu
- 2 soft•boiled eggs, halved
- 2 green onions, sliced
- Sesame seeds for garnish

Instructions:

1. In a large pot, whisk together the broth, miso paste, soy sauce, sesame oil, garlic, and ginger. Bring to a simmer over medium heat.

2. Add the ramen noodles and cook for 2•3 minutes until tender.

3. Stir in the sliced mushrooms and shredded chicken or tofu.

4. Ladle the ramen into bowls and top each serving with a soft•boiled egg, sliced green onions, and a sprinkle of sesame seeds.

5. Serve hot and enjoy!

This miso ramen recipe uses more affordable and accessible ingredients that would be suitable for a teen audience. The miso broth provides a rich, savory flavor, while the mushrooms, chicken/tofu, and soft•boiled egg add protein and heartiness. Please let me know if you would like me to suggest any other teen•friendly ramen recipes.

59. Saffron Ramen

Ingredient:

• 4 cups chicken or vegetable broth
• 1 teaspoon saffron threads
• 2 tablespoons soy sauce
• 1 tablespoon mirin or rice vinegar
• 1 teaspoon sesame oil
• 2 garlic cloves, minced
• 1 inch ginger, grated
• 8 oz ramen noodles
• 1 cup sliced mushrooms
• 1 cup shredded cooked chicken or tofu
• 2 soft•boiled eggs, halved
• 2 green onions, sliced
• Sesame seeds for garnish

Instructions:

1. In a large pot, bring the broth to a simmer over medium heat. Add the saffron threads and let steep for 5 minutes to infuse the broth with the vibrant yellow•orange color and earthy, floral flavor.

2. Stir in the soy sauce, mirin, sesame oil, garlic, and ginger.

3. Add the ramen noodles and cook for 2•3 minutes until tender.

4. Remove from heat and stir in the sliced mushrooms and shredded chicken or tofu.

5. Ladle the ramen into bowls and top each serving with a soft•boiled egg, sliced green onions, and a sprinkle of sesame seeds.

6. Serve hot and enjoy!

The saffron adds a beautiful color and subtle, complex flavor to the ramen broth. The mushrooms, chicken/tofu, and soft•boiled egg provide heartiness and protein, making this a satisfying yet still teen•friendly dish.

Saffron is a premium spice, but a little goes a long way. This recipe uses just a small amount to infuse the broth, keeping the cost reasonable. You can adjust the amount of saffron to your taste preference.

60. Ginger Scallion Ramen

Ingredient:

• 4 cups chicken or vegetable broth
• 2 tablespoons soy sauce
• 1 tablespoon rice vinegar
• 1 teaspoon sesame oil
• 3 tablespoons grated fresh ginger
• 1 cup thinly sliced scallions, plus more for garnish
• 8 oz ramen noodles
• 2 cups shredded cooked chicken or tofu
• 2 soft•boiled eggs, halved
• Sesame seeds for garnish

Instructions:

1. In a large pot, bring the broth, soy sauce, rice vinegar, and sesame oil to a simmer over medium heat.

2. Add the grated ginger and sliced scallions. Simmer for 2•3 minutes to infuse the broth.

3. Add the ramen noodles and cook for 2•3 minutes until tender.

4. Remove from heat and stir in the shredded chicken or tofu.

5. Ladle the ramen into bowls and top each serving with a soft•boiled egg, additional sliced scallions, and a sprinkle of sesame seeds.

6. Serve hot and enjoy!

The ginger and scallions provide a bright, aromatic flavor to the ramen broth. The shredded chicken or tofu adds protein, while the soft•boiled egg provides a rich, creamy element. This recipe is simple, flavorful, and suitable for a teen audience.

You can use either chicken or vegetable broth as the base, depending on your preference. The ginger and scallions are the stars of this dish, so be generous with those ingredients.

61. Spring Vegetable Ramen

Ingredient:

• 4 cups vegetable or chicken broth
• 2 tablespoons soy sauce
• 1 tablespoon mirin or rice vinegar
• 1 teaspoon sesame oil
• 2 garlic cloves, minced
• 1 inch ginger, grated
• 8 oz ramen noodles
• 1 cup sliced asparagus
• 1 cup shelled peas (fresh or frozen)
• 1 cup sliced shiitake mushrooms
• 1 cup shredded cooked chicken or tofu (optional)
• 2 soft•boiled eggs, halved
• 2 green onions, sliced
• Sesame seeds for garnish

Instructions:

1. In a large pot, bring the broth, soy sauce, mirin, sesame oil, garlic, and ginger to a simmer over medium heat.

2. Add the ramen noodles and cook for 2•3 minutes until tender.

3. Stir in the sliced asparagus, shelled peas, and sliced shiitake mushrooms. Cook for 2•3 minutes more until the vegetables are tender•crisp.

4. If using, stir in the shredded chicken or tofu. Ladle the spring vegetable ramen into bowls and top each serving with a soft•boiled egg, sliced green onions, and a sprinkle of sesame seeds. Serve hot and enjoy!

This spring vegetable ramen celebrates the fresh, vibrant produce of the season. The asparagus, peas, and shiitake mushrooms add color, texture, and flavor to the savory broth.

The soft•boiled egg provides a rich, creamy element, while the green onions and sesame seeds offer freshness and crunch. You can also add shredded chicken or tofu for extra protein.

This recipe is vegetarian•friendly, but you can use chicken broth if preferred. Feel free to adjust the vegetable amounts based on your personal tastes.

62. Summer Ramen with Fresh Herbs

Ingredient:

• 4 cups chicken or vegetable broth
• 2 tablespoons soy sauce
• 1 tablespoon rice vinegar
• 1 teaspoon sesame oil
• 2 garlic cloves, minced
• 1 inch ginger, grated
• 8 oz ramen noodles
• 1 cup sliced zucchini or summer squash
• 1 cup shredded cooked chicken or tofu
• 1/2 cup fresh basil leaves
• 1/2 cup fresh cilantro leaves
• 2 soft•boiled eggs, halved
• 2 green onions, sliced
• Lime wedges for serving

Instructions:

1. In a large pot, bring the broth, soy sauce, rice vinegar, and sesame oil to a simmer over medium heat. Stir in the garlic and ginger.

2. Add the ramen noodles and cook for 2•3 minutes until tender.

3. Stir in the sliced zucchini or summer squash and the shredded chicken or tofu. Cook for 1•2 minutes more.

4. Remove from heat and stir in the fresh basil and cilantro leaves.

5. Ladle the ramen into bowls and top each serving with a soft•boiled egg, sliced green onions, and a squeeze of fresh lime juice. Serve hot and enjoy!

The fresh herbs • basil and cilantro • add a bright, summery flavor to this ramen dish. The zucchini or summer squash provides a crisp, seasonal vegetable element.

The soft•boiled egg and lime juice add richness and acidity to balance the savory broth. This ramen is light and refreshing, perfect for enjoying on a warm summer day.

You can use either chicken or vegetable broth as the base, depending on your preference. Tofu is a great vegetarian protein option. Feel free to adjust the herb amounts to your taste.

63. Autumn Pumpkin Ramen

Ingredient:

• 4 cups chicken or vegetable broth
• 1 cup pumpkin puree
• 2 tablespoons soy sauce
• 1 tablespoon mirin or rice vinegar
• 1 teaspoon sesame oil
• 1 teaspoon ground cinnamon
• 1/2 teaspoon ground ginger
• 1/4 teaspoon ground nutmeg
• 2 garlic cloves, minced
• 8 oz ramen noodles
• 1 cup cubed roasted pumpkin or butternut squash
• 1 cup shredded cooked chicken or tofu
• 2 soft•boiled eggs, halved
• 2 green onions, sliced
• Toasted pumpkin seeds for garnish

Instructions:

1. In a large pot, whisk together the broth, pumpkin puree, soy sauce, mirin, sesame oil, cinnamon, ginger, nutmeg, and garlic. Bring to a simmer over medium heat.

2. Add the ramen noodles and cook for 2•3 minutes until tender.

3. Stir in the cubed roasted pumpkin or butternut squash and the shredded chicken or tofu.

4. Ladle the pumpkin ramen into bowls and top each serving with a soft•boiled egg, sliced green onions, and a sprinkle of toasted pumpkin seeds. Serve hot and enjoy!

The pumpkin puree and warm autumn spices create a rich, creamy, and comforting broth that's perfect for the fall season. The roasted pumpkin or squash adds a lovely texture and sweetness.

You can use either chicken or vegetable broth as the base, depending on your preference. Tofu is a great vegetarian protein option.

The soft•boiled egg, green onions, and toasted pumpkin seeds provide contrasting flavors and textures to balance out the pumpkin•forward ramen.

64. Winter Spicy Ramen

Ingredient:

• 4 cups chicken or vegetable broth
• 2 tablespoons gochujang (Korean red chili paste)
• 1 tablespoon soy sauce
• 1 tablespoon mirin or rice vinegar
• 1 teaspoon sesame oil
• 2 garlic cloves, minced
• 1 inch ginger, grated
• 8 oz ramen noodles
• 1 cup sliced shiitake mushrooms
• 1 cup shredded rotisserie chicken or tofu
• 2 soft•boiled eggs, halved
• 2 green onions, sliced
• Sesame seeds for garnish

Instructions:

1. In a large pot, whisk together the broth, gochujang, soy sauce, mirin, sesame oil, garlic, and ginger. Bring to a simmer over medium heat.

2. Add the ramen noodles and cook for 2•3 minutes until tender.

3. Stir in the sliced shiitake mushrooms and shredded chicken or tofu.

4. Ladle the spicy ramen into bowls and top each serving with a soft•boiled egg, sliced green onions, and a sprinkle of sesame seeds.

5. Serve hot and enjoy!

The gochujang (Korean red chili paste) adds a bold, spicy kick to the savory ramen broth, perfect for warming up on a cold winter day. The shiitake mushrooms and chicken or tofu provide heartiness and protein.

The soft•boiled egg adds a rich, creamy element, while the green onions and sesame seeds offer freshness and crunch. This winter spicy ramen is a comforting and flavorful dish.

You can adjust the amount of gochujang to control the spice level, depending on your preference. Vegetable broth can be used instead of chicken for a vegetarian/vegan option.

65. Holiday Ramen

Ingredient:

- 4 cups chicken or vegetable broth
- 2 tablespoons soy sauce
- 1 tablespoon mirin or rice vinegar
- 1 teaspoon sesame oil
- 2 garlic cloves, minced
- 1 inch ginger, grated
- 8 oz ramen noodles
- 1 cup shredded roasted turkey or chicken
- 1 cup steamed broccoli florets
- 1 cup sliced shiitake mushrooms
- 2 soft•boiled eggs, halved
- 2 green onions, sliced
- Cranberry relish or sauce for serving
- Toasted almond slivers for garnish

Instructions:

1. In a large pot, bring the broth, soy sauce, mirin, sesame oil, garlic, and ginger to a simmer over medium heat.

2. Add the ramen noodles and cook for 2•3 minutes until tender.

3. Stir in the shredded roasted turkey or chicken, steamed broccoli florets, and sliced shiitake mushrooms. Cook for 1•2 minutes more.

4. Ladle the holiday ramen into bowls and top each serving with a soft•boiled egg, sliced green onions, a dollop of cranberry relish or sauce, and a sprinkle of toasted almond slivers. Serve hot and enjoy!

This holiday ramen combines classic festive flavors with the comforting elements of a ramen bowl. The shredded turkey or chicken, broccoli, and mushrooms make it a hearty, nourishing meal.

The cranberry relish or sauce adds a sweet•tart contrast, while the toasted almonds provide a nice crunch. The soft•boiled egg and green onions round out the dish.

You can use either chicken or vegetable broth as the base, depending on your preference. Tofu can be substituted for the turkey/chicken for a vegetarian option.

66. New Year's Ramen

Ingredient:

- 4 cups chicken or vegetable broth
- 2 tablespoons soy sauce
- 1 tablespoon mirin or rice vinegar
- 1 teaspoon sesame oil
- 2 garlic cloves, minced
- 1 inch ginger, grated
- 8 oz ramen noodles
- 1 cup shredded roast pork or char siu
- 1 cup shredded cabbage or bok choy
- 1 cup sliced shiitake mushrooms
- 2 soft•boiled eggs, halved
- 2 green onions, sliced
- Toasted sesame seeds for garnish
- Pickled ginger for serving (optional)

Instructions:

1. In a large pot, bring the broth, soy sauce, mirin, sesame oil, garlic, and ginger to a simmer over medium heat.

2. Add the ramen noodles and cook for 2•3 minutes until tender.

3. Stir in the shredded roast pork or char siu, shredded cabbage or bok choy, and sliced shiitake mushrooms. Cook for 1•2 minutes more.

4. Ladle the New Year's ramen into bowls and top each serving with a soft•boiled egg, sliced green onions, and a sprinkle of toasted sesame seeds. Serve hot, with pickled ginger on the side if desired.

This New Year's ramen celebrates the flavors of traditional Asian cuisine, perfect for ringing in the new year. The shredded pork or char siu provides heartiness, while the cabbage/bok choy and mushrooms add freshness and texture.

The soft•boiled egg, green onions, and sesame seeds offer contrasting flavors and elements. The optional pickled ginger adds a bright, tangy note. You can use either chicken or vegetable broth as the base. Tofu can be substituted for the pork/char siu for a vegetarian option.

This New Year's ramen is a delicious and auspicious way to start the new year. The noodles symbolize long life, while the other ingredients represent prosperity and good fortune. Enjoy!

67. Valentine's Day Ramen

Ingredient:

• 4 cups chicken or vegetable broth
• 2 tablespoons soy sauce
• 1 tablespoon mirin or rice vinegar
• 1 teaspoon sesame oil
• 2 garlic cloves, minced
• 1 inch ginger, grated
• 8 oz ramen noodles
• 1 cup sliced mushrooms
• 1 cup shredded cooked chicken or tofu
• 2 soft•boiled eggs, halved
• 2 green onions, sliced
• Heart•shaped sliced beets or radishes for garnish
• Sesame seeds for garnish

Instructions:

1. In a large pot, bring the broth, soy sauce, mirin, sesame oil, garlic, and ginger to a simmer over medium heat.

2. Add the ramen noodles and cook for 2•3 minutes until tender.

3. Remove from heat and stir in the sliced mushrooms and shredded chicken or tofu.

4. Ladle the ramen into bowls and top each serving with a soft•boiled egg, sliced green onions, heart•shaped beet or radish slices, and a sprinkle of sesame seeds.

5. Serve hot and enjoy!

The heart•shaped beet or radish slices add a festive, Valentine's Day touch to this ramen dish. The bright pink color contrasts beautifully with the other ingredients.

This recipe uses accessible, teen•friendly ingredients like chicken or tofu, mushrooms, and soft•boiled eggs. The ramen broth is savory and comforting, making this a wholesome and satisfying meal.

This Valentine's Day ramen would be a fun and creative way to celebrate the holiday with teens. The presentation is visually appealing without being overly indulgent or complicated.

68. St. Patrick's Day Ramen

Ingredient:

• 8 oz ramen noodles
• 4 cups chicken or vegetable broth
• 1 tbsp green curry paste
• 1 tsp honey
• 1 cup shredded cabbage
• 1 cup sliced mushrooms
• 1 cup baby spinach
• 1 green bell pepper, julienned
• 2 green onions, sliced
• 2 soft boiled eggs, halved
• Crushed roasted peanuts for garnish

Instructions:

1. In a large pot, bring the broth to a simmer over medium heat. Whisk in the green curry paste and honey until fully incorporated.

2. Add the ramen noodles and cook according to package instructions, about 3•5 minutes.

3. Stir in the cabbage, mushrooms, spinach, and bell pepper. Cook for 2•3 minutes until the vegetables are tender•crisp.

4. Remove from heat and stir in the green onions.

5. Ladle the St. Patrick's Day ramen into bowls. Top each serving with a soft boiled egg and a sprinkle of crushed roasted peanuts.

6. Serve hot and enjoy the vibrant green colors and flavors of this festive ramen dish!

The green curry paste, cabbage, spinach, and bell pepper give this ramen a fun, St. Patrick's Day•inspired look and flavor. The soft boiled egg and peanuts add texture and richness. This would be a great meal for teens to enjoy on St. Patrick's Day. Adjust the amount of curry paste to your desired spice level.

69. Fourth of July Ramen

Ingredient:

• 8 oz ramen noodles
• 4 cups chicken or vegetable broth
• 1 cup shredded rotisserie chicken
• 1 cup sliced strawberries
• 1 cup blueberries
• 1 cup julienned cucumber
• 2 soft boiled eggs, halved
• 2 tbsp chopped fresh parsley
• Salt and pepper to taste

Instructions:

1. Bring the broth to a boil in a large pot. Add the ramen noodles and cook according to package instructions, about 3•5 minutes.

2. Remove from heat and stir in the shredded chicken.

3. Divide the ramen and broth between 4 bowls.

4. Top each bowl with sliced strawberries, blueberries, and julienned cucumber to create a patriotic red, white, and blue color scheme.

5. Add a soft boiled egg half to each bowl.

6. Sprinkle the chopped parsley over the top for a fresh, herbal garnish.

7. Season with salt and pepper to taste.

8. Serve hot and enjoy this festive Fourth of July ramen!

The combination of the savory chicken, sweet berries, and crunchy cucumber makes for a fun and flavorful ramen dish perfect for celebrating Independence Day. The soft boiled egg adds richness, while the parsley brightens up the flavors. This would be a great meal for teens to enjoy on the Fourth of July. Feel free to adjust the ingredient amounts to your liking.

70. Halloween Ramen

Ingredient:

- 8 oz ramen noodles
- 4 cups chicken or vegetable broth
- 1 cup shredded rotisserie chicken
- 1 cup sliced shiitake mushrooms
- 1 cup shredded purple cabbage
- 1 cup baby spinach
- 2 soft boiled eggs, halved
- 2 tbsp toasted pumpkin seeds
- 1 tsp sesame oil
- Salt and pepper to taste

Instructions:

1. Bring the broth to a boil in a large pot. Add the ramen noodles and cook according to package instructions, about 3•5 minutes.

2. Stir in the shredded chicken, shiitake mushrooms, purple cabbage, and baby spinach. Cook for 2•3 minutes until the vegetables are tender•crisp.

3. Remove from heat and drizzle in the sesame oil. Toss gently to coat.

4. Ladle the Halloween ramen into bowls. Top each serving with a soft boiled egg half and a sprinkle of toasted pumpkin seeds.

5. Season with salt and pepper to taste.

6. Serve hot and enjoy this spooky and delicious ramen!

The purple cabbage and black shiitake mushrooms give this ramen a fun, Halloween•inspired color palette. The shredded chicken, soft boiled egg, and pumpkin seeds provide protein and texture. The sesame oil adds a savory, nutty flavor. This would be a great meal for teens to enjoy around Halloween time. Feel free to adjust the ingredient amounts to your liking.

71. Chicken Nugget Ramen

Ingredient:

• 4 cups chicken broth
• 2 tablespoons soy sauce
• 1 tablespoon mirin or rice vinegar
• 1 teaspoon sesame oil
• 2 garlic cloves, minced
• 1 inch ginger, grated
• 8 oz ramen noodles
• 12•16 frozen chicken nuggets, cooked according to package instructions
• 1 cup shredded cabbage or bok choy
• 2 green onions, sliced
• Sesame seeds for garnish

Instructions:

1. In a large pot, bring the chicken broth, soy sauce, mirin, sesame oil, garlic, and ginger to a simmer over medium heat.

2. Add the ramen noodles and cook for 2•3 minutes until tender.

3. While the noodles are cooking, prepare the chicken nuggets according to the package instructions. Once cooked, slice or break the nuggets into bite•sized pieces.

4. Stir the shredded cabbage or bok choy into the ramen broth and cook for 1•2 minutes until slightly wilted.

5. Remove from heat and stir in the sliced chicken nuggets.

6. Ladle the chicken nugget ramen into bowls and top with sliced green onions and a sprinkle of sesame seeds. Serve hot and enjoy!

This chicken nugget ramen is a fun and creative twist on a classic ramen dish. The crispy, breaded chicken nuggets add a satisfying texture and flavor to the savory broth.

The cabbage or bok choy provides a fresh, crunchy element, while the green onions and sesame seeds offer additional flavor and garnish. You can use any brand of frozen chicken nuggets for this recipe. Adjust the amount based on your personal preference. This dish is sure to be a hit with kids and adults alike!

72. Mac and Cheese Ramen

Ingredient:

- 4 cups chicken or vegetable broth
- 1 cup milk
- 2 tablespoons butter
- 2 tablespoons all•purpose flour
- 1 cup shredded cheddar cheese
- 1/2 cup grated parmesan cheese
- 1/2 teaspoon garlic powder
- 1/2 teaspoon onion powder
- 1/4 teaspoon cayenne pepper (optional)
- 8 oz ramen noodles
- 2 green onions, sliced
- Crispy fried onions or panko breadcrumbs for garnish (optional)

Instructions:

1. In a large pot, bring the broth and milk to a simmer over medium heat.

2. In a separate saucepan, melt the butter over medium heat. Whisk in the flour and cook for 1•2 minutes to make a roux.

3. Gradually whisk the roux into the simmering broth and milk mixture. Cook for 2•3 minutes until thickened.

4. Remove from heat and stir in the shredded cheddar, grated parmesan, garlic powder, onion powder, and cayenne (if using) until the cheese is melted and the sauce is smooth.

5. Add the ramen noodles to the cheese sauce and cook for 2•3 minutes until the noodles are tender.

6. Ladle the mac and cheese ramen into bowls and top with sliced green onions and crispy fried onions or panko breadcrumbs, if desired. Serve hot and enjoy!

This mac and cheese ramen combines the comfort of classic mac and cheese with the slurpable noodles of ramen. The creamy, cheesy sauce coats the ramen noodles for a truly indulgent dish.

You can use either chicken or vegetable broth as the base. The cayenne pepper adds a subtle kick, but it's optional if you prefer a milder flavor.

The crispy fried onions or panko breadcrumbs provide a nice textural contrast to the soft noodles and creamy sauce. This mac and cheese ramen makes for a satisfying and comforting meal.

73. Pizza Ramen

Ingredient:

• 8 oz ramen noodles
• 4 cups tomato or marinara sauce
• 1 tsp dried oregano
• 1/2 tsp garlic powder
• 1/4 tsp red pepper flakes (optional)
• 1 cup shredded mozzarella cheese
• 1/2 cup sliced pepperoni
• 1/2 cup sliced mushrooms
• 1/2 cup diced bell pepper
• 2 green onions, sliced
• Grated Parmesan cheese for serving

Instructions:

1. In a large pot, bring the tomato or marinara sauce to a simmer over medium heat. Stir in the dried oregano, garlic powder, and red pepper flakes (if using).

2. Add the ramen noodles and cook according to package instructions, about 3•5 minutes.

3. Remove from heat and stir in the shredded mozzarella cheese until melted and well combined.

4. Divide the pizza ramen between bowls. Top each serving with sliced pepperoni, mushrooms, bell pepper, and green onions.

5. Sprinkle grated Parmesan cheese over the top.

6. Serve hot and enjoy this fun and flavorful pizza•inspired ramen!

This ramen dish captures all the classic flavors of a pepperoni pizza in a comforting noodle bowl. The tomato sauce, oregano, and mozzarella cheese create that familiar pizza taste, while the pepperoni, mushrooms, and bell pepper add texture and variety. This would be a great meal for teens to enjoy. Feel free to adjust the toppings to your liking.

74. Cheeseburger Ramen

Ingredient:

• 8 oz ramen noodles
• 4 cups beef or chicken broth
• 1 lb ground beef
• 1 onion, diced
• 2 cloves garlic, minced
• 2 tbsp tomato paste
• 1 tsp Worcestershire sauce
• 1 tsp dried oregano
• Salt and pepper to taste
• 1 cup shredded cheddar cheese
• 2 soft boiled eggs, halved
• Diced pickles, for serving (optional)

Instructions:

1. In a large skillet, cook the ground beef over medium•high heat, breaking it up as it cooks, until browned and cooked through, about 5•7 minutes. Drain any excess fat.

2. Add the diced onion and minced garlic to the skillet. Cook for 2•3 minutes until the onion is translucent.

3. Stir in the tomato paste, Worcestershire sauce, oregano, salt, and pepper. Cook for 1 minute.

4. Pour in the beef or chicken broth and bring to a boil. Add the ramen noodles and cook according to package instructions, about 3•5 minutes.

5. Remove from heat and stir in the shredded cheddar cheese until melted and well combined.

6. Ladle the cheeseburger ramen into bowls. Top each serving with a soft boiled egg half and diced pickles, if desired. Serve hot and enjoy this fun and flavorful cheeseburger•inspired ramen!

This ramen dish combines the savory, beefy flavors of a cheeseburger with the comfort of ramen noodles. The soft boiled egg and pickles add extra toppings just like a real cheeseburger. This would be a great meal for teens to enjoy. Adjust the cheese and seasoning to your taste preferences.

75. PB&J Ramen

Ingredient:

• 8 oz ramen noodles
• 4 cups chicken or vegetable broth
• 1/4 cup creamy peanut butter
• 2 tbsp strawberry jam
• 1 tbsp soy sauce
• 1 tsp rice vinegar
• 1 tsp honey
• 1 cup sliced strawberries
• 2 tbsp chopped roasted peanuts
• 2 green onions, sliced
• 2 soft boiled eggs, halved (optional)

Instructions:

1. In a medium saucepan, whisk together the broth, peanut butter, strawberry jam, soy sauce, rice vinegar, and honey until smooth and well combined.

2. Bring the broth mixture to a simmer over medium heat. Add the ramen noodles and cook according to package instructions, about 3•5 minutes.

3. Remove from heat and stir in the sliced strawberries.

4. Ladle the PB&J ramen into bowls. Top each serving with chopped roasted peanuts and sliced green onions.

5. If desired, add a soft boiled egg half to each bowl for extra protein and richness.

6. Serve hot and enjoy this unique and tasty PB&J•inspired ramen!

This ramen dish combines the classic flavors of peanut butter and jelly in a fun and creative way. The peanut butter and strawberry jam create a sweet and savory broth, while the fresh strawberries and crunchy peanuts add texture. The soft boiled egg is an optional addition that provides extra protein. This would be a great meal for teens to enjoy. Adjust the amounts of peanut butter and jam to your taste preferences.

76. Sloppy Joe Ramen

Ingredient:

• 8 oz ramen noodles
• 1 lb ground beef
• 1 onion, diced
• 2 cloves garlic, minced
• 1 cup tomato sauce
• 2 tbsp brown sugar
• 2 tbsp Worcestershire sauce
• 1 tsp chili powder
• 1/2 tsp smoked paprika
• Salt and pepper to taste
• 2 cups shredded cabbage
• 2 green onions, sliced
• 2 soft boiled eggs, halved (optional)

Instructions:

1. In a large skillet, cook the ground beef over medium•high heat, breaking it up as it cooks, until browned and cooked through, about 5•7 minutes. Drain any excess fat.

2. Add the diced onion and minced garlic to the skillet. Cook for 2•3 minutes until the onion is translucent.

3. Stir in the tomato sauce, brown sugar, Worcestershire sauce, chili powder, and smoked paprika. Season with salt and pepper to taste. Simmer for 5•10 minutes, allowing the flavors to meld.

4. Meanwhile, bring a pot of water to a boil and cook the ramen noodles according to package instructions, about 3•5 minutes. Drain and set aside.

5. Add the cooked ramen noodles to the sloppy joe mixture and toss to combine. Divide the sloppy joe ramen between bowls. Top each serving with shredded cabbage, sliced green onions, and a soft boiled egg half, if desired. Serve hot and enjoy this messy, but delicious, sloppy joe•inspired ramen!

This ramen dish combines the classic flavors of a sloppy joe with the comfort of ramen noodles. The ground beef, tomato sauce, and spices create a savory, slightly sweet sauce that coats the noodles. The cabbage and green onions add freshness and crunch. The soft boiled egg is an optional addition that provides extra richness. This would be a great meal for teens to enjoy.

77. Spaghetti Ramen

Ingredient:

• 4 cups chicken or vegetable broth
• 1 (14 oz) can diced tomatoes
• 2 tablespoons tomato paste
• 1 teaspoon dried oregano
• 1/2 teaspoon garlic powder
• 1/4 teaspoon crushed red pepper flakes (optional)
• Salt and pepper to taste
• 8 oz ramen noodles
• 1 cup shredded mozzarella cheese
• 1/4 cup grated parmesan cheese
• 2 tablespoons chopped fresh basil
• 2 green onions, sliced

Instructions:

1. In a large pot, combine the broth, diced tomatoes, tomato paste, oregano, garlic powder, and red pepper flakes (if using). Season with salt and pepper. Bring to a simmer over medium heat.

2. Add the ramen noodles and cook for 2•3 minutes until tender.

3. Remove from heat and stir in the shredded mozzarella and parmesan cheeses until melted and creamy.

4. Ladle the spaghetti ramen into bowls and top with chopped fresh basil and sliced green onions. Serve hot and enjoy!

This spaghetti ramen dish combines the flavors of classic Italian pasta with the slurpable noodles of ramen. The tomato•based broth provides a savory, saucy element, while the melted cheeses add richness and creaminess.

You can use either chicken or vegetable broth as the base. The red pepper flakes add a subtle heat, but they're optional if you prefer a milder flavor. The fresh basil and green onions offer a bright, herbal contrast to the tomato•cheese sauce. This spaghetti ramen makes for a comforting and satisfying meal.

Feel free to customize the toppings or add other Italian•inspired ingredients like ground beef, Italian sausage, or roasted vegetables. Enjoy this unique fusion of pasta and ramen!

78. Corn Dog Ramen

Ingredient:

- 8 oz ramen noodles
- 4 cups chicken or beef broth
- 4 hot dogs, cut into 1•inch pieces
- 1 cup cornmeal
- 1/4 cup all•purpose flour
- 1 tsp baking powder
- 1 tbsp sugar
- 1/2 tsp salt
- 1 egg, beaten
- 2 tbsp milk
- 2 green onions, sliced
- Honey mustard for serving (optional)

Instructions:

1. In a large pot, bring the broth to a boil over high heat. Add the ramen noodles and cook according to package instructions, about 3•5 minutes.

2. In a shallow bowl, combine the cornmeal, flour, baking powder, sugar, and salt.

3. In a separate bowl, whisk together the beaten egg and milk.

4. Dip the hot dog pieces into the egg mixture, then coat them in the cornmeal mixture, pressing to adhere.

5. Carefully add the coated hot dog pieces to the boiling ramen broth. Reduce heat to medium and cook for 5•7 minutes, until the cornmeal coating is golden brown and crispy.

6. Remove from heat and stir in the sliced green onions.

7. Ladle the corn dog ramen into bowls. Serve with honey mustard for dipping, if desired.

8. Enjoy this fun and tasty corn dog•inspired ramen!

This ramen dish puts a creative spin on the classic corn dog. The cornmeal•coated hot dog pieces add a fun, crunchy texture to the savory broth and noodles. The green onions provide a fresh contrast. This would be a great meal for teens to enjoy. Feel free to adjust the seasoning or add any other desired toppings.

79. Hot Dog Ramen

Ingredient:

• 8 oz ramen noodles
• 4 cups chicken or beef broth
• 4 hot dogs, sliced into rounds
• 1 cup shredded cabbage
• 1 carrot, julienned
• 2 green onions, sliced
• 2 tbsp ketchup
• 1 tbsp yellow mustard
• 1 tsp brown sugar
• Salt and pepper to taste
• Crushed potato chips for garnish (optional)

Instructions:

1. In a large pot, bring the broth to a boil over high heat. Add the ramen noodles and cook according to package instructions, about 3•5 minutes.

2. Reduce heat to medium and stir in the sliced hot dogs, shredded cabbage, and julienned carrot. Cook for 2•3 minutes until the vegetables are tender•crisp.

3. In a small bowl, whisk together the ketchup, mustard, and brown sugar. Pour this sauce into the ramen pot and stir to coat the ingredients.

4. Remove from heat and stir in the sliced green onions. Season with salt and pepper to taste.

5. Ladle the hot dog ramen into bowls. Top each serving with a sprinkle of crushed potato chips, if desired.

6. Serve hot and enjoy this fun and flavorful ramen twist on a classic hot dog!

This ramen dish captures all the classic flavors of a hot dog, from the savory sausage to the sweet and tangy condiments. The crunchy cabbage, carrot, and potato chips add great texture. This would be a great meal for teens to enjoy. Feel free to adjust the amount of ketchup, mustard, and brown sugar to your taste preferences.

80. Meatball Ramen

Ingredient:

- 8 oz ramen noodles
- 4 cups chicken or beef broth
- 1 lb ground beef
- 1/2 cup breadcrumbs
- 1 egg
- 2 cloves garlic, minced
- 1 tsp dried oregano
- Salt and pepper to taste
- 1 cup sliced mushrooms
- 1 cup baby spinach
- 2 green onions, sliced
- Grated Parmesan cheese for serving (optional)

Instructions:

1. In a medium bowl, combine the ground beef, breadcrumbs, egg, minced garlic, dried oregano, salt, and pepper. Mix well until fully incorporated.

2. Roll the beef mixture into small, bite•sized meatballs, about 1•inch in size.

3. In a large pot, bring the broth to a simmer over medium heat. Carefully add the meatballs to the simmering broth and cook for 8•10 minutes, until the meatballs are cooked through.

4. Add the ramen noodles to the pot and cook according to package instructions, about 3•5 minutes.

5. Stir in the sliced mushrooms and baby spinach. Cook for 2•3 minutes until the vegetables are tender.

6. Remove from heat and stir in the sliced green onions. Ladle the meatball ramen into bowls. Top with grated Parmesan cheese, if desired. Serve hot and enjoy this hearty and comforting meatball ramen!

This ramen dish combines the classic flavors of meatballs and marinara with the comfort of ramen noodles. The meatballs provide a satisfying protein, while the mushrooms, spinach, and green onions add freshness and texture. This would be a great meal for teens to enjoy. Feel free to adjust the seasoning or add any other desired toppings.

81. Chocolate Ramen

Ingredient:

• 8 oz ramen noodles
• 4 cups milk
• 1/2 cup unsweetened cocoa powder
• 1/4 cup granulated sugar
• 1 tsp vanilla extract
• Pinch of salt
• 1 cup mini marshmallows
• Whipped cream for serving (optional)
• Crushed graham crackers for garnish (optional)

Instructions:

1. In a large saucepan, whisk together the milk, cocoa powder, sugar, vanilla, and salt over medium heat. Bring the mixture to a gentle simmer, whisking frequently, until the sugar has dissolved and the cocoa is fully incorporated, about 5 minutes.

2. Add the ramen noodles to the pot and cook according to package instructions, about 3•5 minutes.

3. Remove from heat and stir in the mini marshmallows until they are melted and the mixture is smooth.

4. Ladle the chocolate ramen into bowls.

5. Top each serving with a dollop of whipped cream and a sprinkle of crushed graham crackers, if desired.

6. Serve hot and enjoy this decadent and indulgent chocolate ramen!

This ramen dish puts a sweet and creative twist on the classic savory preparation. The rich chocolate broth, melted marshmallows, and optional toppings make this a truly unique and indulgent treat. While it may be a bit more dessert•like, this chocolate ramen could still be a fun and suitable option for teens to enjoy. Adjust the amount of sugar to your taste preference.

82. Strawberry Ramen

Ingredient:

• 8 oz ramen noodles
• 4 cups strawberry juice or puree
• 1/4 cup granulated sugar
• 1 tsp vanilla extract
• 1 cup sliced fresh strawberries
• 2 tbsp chopped fresh basil (optional)
• Whipped cream for serving (optional)

Instructions:

1. In a large saucepan, combine the strawberry juice or puree, sugar, and vanilla extract. Bring the mixture to a simmer over medium heat, stirring occasionally, until the sugar has dissolved, about 5 minutes.

2. Add the ramen noodles to the pot and cook according to package instructions, about 3•5 minutes.

3. Remove from heat and stir in the sliced fresh strawberries.

4. Ladle the strawberry ramen into bowls.

5. Top each serving with a dollop of whipped cream and a sprinkle of chopped fresh basil, if desired.

6. Serve hot and enjoy this sweet and fruity ramen!

This ramen dish features a vibrant strawberry•flavored broth that is both sweet and refreshing. The fresh strawberries add a nice texture and burst of flavor. The optional whipped cream and basil garnish provide a nice contrast.

This would be a fun and creative ramen option that would be suitable for teens. The sweetness and bright color make it an appealing and unique dish. Adjust the amount of sugar to your taste preference. You could also try using a strawberry puree or jam for a thicker, more intense strawberry flavor.

83. Mango Ramen

Ingredient:

• 8 oz ramen noodles
• 4 cups chicken or vegetable broth
• 1 ripe mango, peeled and diced
• 1 cup shredded cooked chicken
• 1 cup shredded red cabbage
• 1 cup sliced cucumber
• 2 green onions, sliced
• 1 tbsp rice vinegar
• 1 tsp sesame oil
• Salt and pepper to taste
• Chopped cilantro for garnish (optional)

Instructions:

1. Bring the broth to a boil in a large pot. Add the ramen noodles and cook according to package instructions, about 3•5 minutes.

2. Remove from heat and stir in the diced mango, shredded chicken, red cabbage, and sliced cucumber.

3. In a small bowl, whisk together the rice vinegar and sesame oil. Drizzle this dressing over the ramen and toss gently to coat.

4. Season with salt and pepper to taste.

5. Ladle the mango ramen into bowls and top with sliced green onions and chopped cilantro, if desired.

6. Serve hot and enjoy the sweet, tangy, and refreshing flavors of this mango ramen!

This ramen dish features the bright, tropical flavors of mango paired with savory chicken and crunchy vegetables. The rice vinegar and sesame oil dressing adds a nice balance of acidity and nuttiness. This would be a great meal for teens to enjoy, as the mango provides a fun, fruity twist on traditional ramen. Feel free to adjust the ingredient amounts to your taste preferences.

84. Blueberry Ramen

Ingredient:

- 8 oz ramen noodles
- 4 cups blueberry juice or puree
- 1/4 cup honey
- 1 tsp lemon zest
- 1 cup fresh blueberries
- 2 tbsp chopped fresh mint (optional)
- Whipped cream for serving (optional)

Instructions:

1. In a large saucepan, combine the blueberry juice or puree, honey, and lemon zest. Bring the mixture to a simmer over medium heat, stirring occasionally, until the honey has dissolved, about 5 minutes.

2. Add the ramen noodles to the pot and cook according to package instructions, about 3-5 minutes.

3. Remove from heat and stir in the fresh blueberries.

4. Ladle the blueberry ramen into bowls.

5. Top each serving with a dollop of whipped cream and a sprinkle of chopped fresh mint, if desired.

6. Serve hot and enjoy this vibrant and fruity blueberry ramen!

This ramen dish features a rich, blueberry-infused broth that is sweetened with honey and brightened with lemon zest. The fresh blueberries add a nice texture and burst of flavor. The optional whipped cream and mint garnish provide a nice contrast.

This would be a fun and creative ramen option that would be suitable for teens. The deep purple color and sweet-tart flavor profile make it an appealing and unique dish. Adjust the amount of honey to your taste preference. You could also try using a blueberry puree for a thicker, more intense blueberry flavor.

85. Pumpkin Spice Ramen

Ingredient:

• 8 oz ramen noodles
• 4 cups chicken or vegetable broth
• 1 cup pumpkin puree
• 1/4 cup heavy cream
• 2 tbsp brown sugar
• 1 tsp pumpkin pie spice
• 1/2 tsp ground cinnamon
• 1/4 tsp ground ginger
• 1/4 tsp ground nutmeg
• Salt and pepper to taste
• Toasted pumpkin seeds for garnish (optional)
• Whipped cream for serving (optional)

Instructions:

1. In a large saucepan, whisk together the broth, pumpkin puree, heavy cream, brown sugar, pumpkin pie spice, cinnamon, ginger, and nutmeg. Bring the mixture to a simmer over medium heat, stirring occasionally, until well combined and slightly thickened, about 5•7 minutes.

2. Add the ramen noodles to the pot and cook according to package instructions, about 3•5 minutes.

3. Remove from heat and season with salt and pepper to taste.

4. Ladle the pumpkin spice ramen into bowls.

5. Top each serving with a sprinkle of toasted pumpkin seeds and a dollop of whipped cream, if desired. Serve hot and enjoy this cozy and autumnal pumpkin spice ramen!

This ramen dish captures all the warm, comforting flavors of pumpkin pie in a savory noodle bowl. The pumpkin puree, heavy cream, and blend of spices create a rich, creamy broth that pairs perfectly with the ramen noodles. The toasted pumpkin seeds and optional whipped cream add texture and extra creaminess.

This pumpkin spice ramen would be a fun and seasonal option that would be suitable for teens. The vibrant orange color and festive flavors make it an appealing and unique dish. Adjust the spice blend to your taste preference.

86. Lavender Ramen

Ingredient:

• 8 oz ramen noodles
• 4 cups chicken or vegetable broth
• 2 tbsp dried lavender flowers
• 2 tsp honey
• 1 tsp soy sauce
• 1 cup shredded chicken or tofu
• 2 soft boiled eggs, halved
• 2 green onions, sliced
• Salt and pepper to taste

Instructions:

1. In a medium saucepan, bring the broth to a boil over high heat. Reduce heat to low and stir in the dried lavender flowers. Simmer for 5•10 minutes to infuse the broth with lavender flavor.

2. Strain the broth through a fine mesh sieve to remove the lavender flowers. Return the broth to the pan and stir in the honey and soy sauce. Taste and adjust seasoning as needed.

3. Add the ramen noodles to the broth and cook according to package instructions, about 3•5 minutes.

4. Remove from heat and stir in the shredded chicken or tofu.

5. Ladle the lavender ramen into bowls. Top each serving with a soft boiled egg, sliced green onions, and a sprinkle of salt and pepper.

6. Serve hot and enjoy the soothing, floral notes of the lavender ramen!

The lavender adds a lovely, aromatic flavor to the broth that pairs beautifully with the savory ramen. Feel free to adjust the amount of lavender to your taste preference. Enjoy this unique and comforting ramen dish!

87. Matcha Ramen

Ingredient:

• 8 oz ramen noodles
• 4 cups chicken or vegetable broth
• 2 tsp matcha green tea powder
• 1 tbsp honey
• 1 tsp soy sauce
• 1 cup shredded chicken or tofu
• 2 soft boiled eggs, halved
• 2 green onions, sliced
• Sesame seeds for garnish

Instructions:

1. In a medium saucepan, whisk together the broth, matcha powder, honey, and soy sauce. Bring to a simmer over medium heat, whisking occasionally, until the matcha is fully dissolved.

2. Add the ramen noodles to the broth and cook according to package instructions, about 3•5 minutes.

3. Remove from heat and stir in the shredded chicken or tofu.

4. Ladle the matcha ramen into bowls. Top each serving with a soft boiled egg, sliced green onions, and a sprinkle of sesame seeds.

5. Serve hot and enjoy the vibrant green color and earthy, slightly sweet flavor of the matcha ramen.

This matcha ramen is a fun and visually appealing dish that would be suitable for teens. The matcha powder provides a boost of antioxidants and a unique flavor profile, while the honey and soy sauce balance it out. The soft boiled egg and protein•rich chicken or tofu make it a satisfying meal. Adjust the amount of matcha to your taste preference. Enjoy!

88. Rainbow Ramen

Ingredient:

- 8 oz ramen noodles
- 4 cups vegetable or chicken broth
- 1 cup shredded cabbage
- 1 carrot, julienned
- 1 bell pepper, sliced
- 1 cup sliced mushrooms
- 2 green onions, sliced
- 1 egg, soft boiled
- Sesame seeds for garnish

Instructions:

1. Bring the broth to a boil in a large pot. Add the ramen noodles and cook according to package instructions, about 3•5 minutes.

2. Add the cabbage, carrot, bell pepper, and mushrooms to the pot. Cook for 2•3 minutes until the vegetables are tender•crisp.

3. Remove from heat and stir in the green onions.

4. Ladle the ramen and vegetables into a bowl. Top with the soft boiled egg and sprinkle with sesame seeds.

5. Serve hot and enjoy your colorful and flavorful Rainbow Ramen!

The key to this dish is using a variety of fresh, vibrant vegetables to create the "rainbow" effect. Feel free to customize the veggies based on your preferences. The soft boiled egg adds a nice richness. Enjoy!

89. Unicorn Ramen

Ingredient:

- 8 oz ramen noodles
- 4 cups chicken or vegetable broth
- 1/2 cup whole milk
- 1/4 cup white chocolate chips
- 1•2 drops blue food coloring
- 1•2 drops pink food coloring
- 1 cup shredded rotisserie chicken
- 1 cup sliced strawberries
- 1 cup blueberries
- Edible glitter or sprinkles (optional)
- Whipped cream for serving (optional)

Instructions:

1. In a medium saucepan, combine the broth and milk. Bring to a gentle simmer over medium heat.

2. Remove from heat and stir in the white chocolate chips until melted and fully incorporated.

3. Divide the broth mixture evenly between two bowls. In one bowl, add 1•2 drops of blue food coloring and stir to combine. In the other bowl, add 1•2 drops of pink food coloring and stir.

4. Add the ramen noodles to the colored broths and cook according to package instructions, about 3•5 minutes.

5. Divide the blue and pink ramen noodles between 4 serving bowls.

6. Top each bowl with shredded rotisserie chicken, sliced strawberries, and blueberries. If desired, sprinkle with edible glitter or sprinkles for a truly magical touch. Serve warm, with a dollop of whipped cream on top.

This Unicorn Ramen is a fun and colorful twist on the classic dish. The white chocolate•infused broth creates a creamy, sweet base that is then divided and colored with blue and pink food dyes. The fresh fruit toppings add pops of color and natural sweetness. The optional edible glitter and whipped cream make this ramen extra magical and whimsical. This would be a great meal for teens to enjoy.

90. Galaxy Ramen

Ingredient:

• 8 oz ramen noodles
• 4 cups chicken or vegetable broth
• 1/4 cup soy sauce
• 2 tbsp rice vinegar
• 1 tbsp sesame oil
• 1 tsp honey
• 1•2 drops each of blue, purple, and black food coloring
• 1 cup shredded rotisserie chicken
• 1 cup sliced mushrooms
• 1 cup shredded purple cabbage
• 2 green onions, sliced
• Toasted sesame seeds for garnish
• Edible glitter or stars (optional)

Instructions:

1. In a large pot, combine the broth, soy sauce, rice vinegar, sesame oil, and honey. Whisk to blend.

2. Add 1•2 drops each of blue, purple, and black food coloring to the broth. Stir gently to create a swirling, galaxy•like effect.

3. Bring the colored broth to a simmer over medium heat. Add the ramen noodles and cook according to package instructions, about 3•5 minutes.

4. Remove from heat and stir in the shredded chicken, sliced mushrooms, and shredded purple cabbage.

5. Ladle the Galaxy Ramen into bowls. Top each serving with sliced green onions and a sprinkle of toasted sesame seeds.

6. For an extra cosmic touch, you can lightly dust the ramen with edible glitter or sprinkle on some edible star•shaped confetti. Serve hot and enjoy this out•of•this•world ramen creation!

The key to this Galaxy Ramen is the colorful, swirling broth that mimics the look of a starry night sky. The combination of blue, purple, and black food coloring creates a dramatic, galactic effect. The toppings of shredded chicken, mushrooms, and purple cabbage add texture and flavor. The edible glitter or stars are an optional, but fun, finishing touch.

91. Tokyo Style Ramen

Ingredient:

• 8 oz ramen noodles
• 4 cups chicken or pork broth
• 2 tbsp soy sauce
• 1 tbsp mirin
• 1 tsp sesame oil
• 1 tsp sugar
• 1/2 tsp ground white pepper
• 1 cup sliced chashu pork (or other braised pork)
• 2 soft boiled eggs, halved
• 1 cup baby spinach
• 2 green onions, sliced
• Nori sheets, cut into strips
• Toasted sesame seeds for garnish

Instructions:

1. In a large pot, combine the broth, soy sauce, mirin, sesame oil, sugar, and white pepper. Bring to a simmer over medium heat.

2. Add the ramen noodles to the pot and cook according to package instructions, about 3•5 minutes.

3. Remove from heat and ladle the Tokyo style ramen into bowls.

4. Top each serving with slices of chashu pork, soft boiled egg halves, baby spinach, sliced green onions, and nori strips.

5. Sprinkle with toasted sesame seeds for garnish. Serve hot and enjoy the authentic flavors of Tokyo•style ramen.

The hallmarks of Tokyo style ramen are the rich, umami•forward broth seasoned with soy sauce, mirin, and white pepper, as well as the tender chashu pork topping. The soft boiled egg, spinach, and green onions add freshness and texture.

This style of ramen is known for its balance of bold, savory flavors and delicate, refined elements. The nori strips and sesame seeds provide the finishing touches that make this Tokyo•inspired ramen truly authentic.

92. Osaka Style Ramen

Ingredient:

• 8 oz ramen noodles
• 4 cups pork or chicken broth
• 2 tbsp takoyaki sauce (or okonomiyaki sauce)
• 1 tbsp Worcestershire sauce
• 1 tsp brown sugar
• 1/2 tsp garlic powder
• 1/2 tsp onion powder
• 1 cup shredded pork or chicken
• 1 cup shredded cabbage
• 2 green onions, sliced
• 1 soft boiled egg, halved
• Pickled ginger for serving (optional)

Instructions:

1. In a large pot, combine the broth, takoyaki sauce, Worcestershire sauce, brown sugar, garlic powder, and onion powder. Bring to a simmer over medium heat.

2. Add the ramen noodles to the pot and cook according to package instructions, about 3•5 minutes.

3. Remove from heat and stir in the shredded pork or chicken and shredded cabbage.

4. Ladle the Osaka style ramen into bowls.

5. Top each serving with a soft boiled egg half, sliced green onions, and a side of pickled ginger, if desired. Serve hot and enjoy the bold, savory flavors of this Osaka•inspired ramen.

The key elements of Osaka style ramen are the use of takoyaki or okonomiyaki sauce, which provides a sweet and tangy flavor profile, as well as the addition of Worcestershire sauce for extra umami. The shredded pork or chicken and cabbage add heartiness and texture.

This ramen would be suitable for teens as the flavors, while bold, are not overly complex or spicy. The soft boiled egg and pickled ginger are optional toppings that can be adjusted to personal preference. Overall, this Osaka style ramen offers a delicious and approachable take on the classic Japanese dish.

93. Kyoto Style Ramen

Ingredient:

• 8 oz ramen noodles
• 4 cups dashi broth (or chicken/vegetable broth)
• 2 tbsp soy sauce
• 1 tbsp mirin
• 1 tsp sugar
• 4 oz thinly sliced pork belly or char siu
• 2 soft boiled eggs, halved
• 1 cup shredded napa cabbage
• 2 green onions, sliced
• 1 sheet of nori, cut into strips
• Toasted sesame seeds for garnish

For the Dashi Broth:
• 4 cups water
• 1 (3•inch) piece kombu (dried kelp)
• 1 cup bonito flakes

Instructions:
Dashi Broth:

1. In a large pot, combine the water and kombu. Let soak for 30 minutes.
2. Bring the pot to a simmer over medium heat and remove the kombu just before it starts to boil.
3. Add the bonito flakes and let steep for 5•10 minutes. Strain the broth through a fine mesh sieve.

Ramen:

1. In a medium saucepan, combine the dashi broth, soy sauce, mirin, and sugar. Bring to a simmer over medium heat.
2. Add the ramen noodles and cook according to package instructions, about 3•5 minutes.
3. Divide the ramen and broth between 4 bowls.
4. Top each bowl with sliced pork belly, soft boiled egg halves, shredded napa cabbage, green onions, nori strips, and a sprinkle of toasted sesame seeds.
5. Serve hot and enjoy the authentic flavors of Kyoto style ramen!

The key to this ramen is the homemade dashi broth, which provides a rich, umami•packed base. The soy sauce, mirin, and sugar create a balanced, savory•sweet flavor profile. The toppings of tender pork, soft boiled egg, crunchy cabbage, and aromatic garnishes make this a truly satisfying and authentic Kyoto•style ramen.

94. Sapporo Style Ramen

Ingredient:

- 8 oz ramen noodles
- 4 cups pork or chicken broth
- 2 tbsp miso paste
- 1 tbsp soy sauce
- 1 tsp sesame oil
- 1/2 tsp ground white pepper
- 1 cup sliced pork belly or chashu pork
- 2 soft boiled eggs, halved
- 1 cup shredded cabbage
- 2 green onions, sliced
- Toasted sesame seeds for garnish

Instructions:

1. In a large pot, whisk together the broth, miso paste, soy sauce, sesame oil, and white pepper until well combined.

2. Bring the miso•flavored broth to a simmer over medium heat.

3. Add the ramen noodles to the pot and cook according to package instructions, about 3•5 minutes.

4. Remove from heat and ladle the Sapporo style ramen into bowls.

5. Top each serving with slices of pork belly or chashu pork, soft boiled egg halves, shredded cabbage, and sliced green onions.

6. Sprinkle with toasted sesame seeds for garnish.

7. Serve hot and enjoy the rich, umami•forward flavors of this Sapporo•inspired ramen.

Sapporo, the capital of Japan's northernmost island of Hokkaido, is known for its hearty, miso•based ramen. The key elements of this style are the use of miso paste to create a bold, savory broth, as well as the tender pork belly or chashu pork topping.

The soft boiled egg, shredded cabbage, and green onions add contrasting textures and freshness to balance out the rich broth. The toasted sesame seeds provide a nutty finishing touch.

95. Hakodate Style Ramen

Ingredient:

• 8 oz ramen noodles
• 4 cups seafood or chicken broth
• 2 tbsp soy sauce
• 1 tbsp mirin
• 1 tsp sesame oil
• 1/2 tsp ground white pepper
• 1 cup cooked shrimp, peeled and deveined
• 1 cup sliced shiitake mushrooms
• 1 cup baby bok choy, chopped
• 2 green onions, sliced
• Toasted sesame seeds for garnish

Instructions:

1. In a large pot, combine the seafood or chicken broth, soy sauce, mirin, sesame oil, and white pepper. Bring to a simmer over medium heat.

2. Add the ramen noodles to the pot and cook according to package instructions, about 3•5 minutes.

3. Stir in the cooked shrimp, sliced shiitake mushrooms, and chopped baby bok choy. Cook for an additional 2•3 minutes until the vegetables are tender.

4. Remove from heat and ladle the Hakodate style ramen into bowls.

5. Top each serving with sliced green onions and a sprinkle of toasted sesame seeds.
Serve hot and enjoy the delicate, seafood•forward flavors of this Hakodate•inspired ramen.

Hakodate is a port city in northern Japan known for its fresh seafood, and this ramen reflects that influence. The broth is seasoned with soy sauce, mirin, and white pepper, creating a light yet flavorful base. The shrimp, shiitake mushrooms, and baby bok choy provide a variety of textures and tastes.

This Hakodate style ramen would be suitable for teens as the flavors are not overpowering, and the dish features familiar ingredients like shrimp and vegetables. The sesame seed garnish adds a nice nutty crunch. Feel free to adjust the protein or vegetable components to your liking.

96. Fukuoka Style Ramen

Ingredient:

• 8 oz ramen noodles
• 4 cups pork bone broth
• 2 tbsp soy sauce
• 1 tbsp mirin
• 1 tsp sesame oil
• 1/2 tsp ground white pepper
• 1 cup thinly sliced pork belly or chashu pork
• 2 soft boiled eggs, halved
• 1 cup bean sprouts
• 2 green onions, sliced
• Pickled ginger for serving (optional)

Instructions:

1. In a large pot, combine the pork bone broth, soy sauce, mirin, sesame oil, and white pepper. Bring to a simmer over medium heat.

2. Add the ramen noodles to the pot and cook according to package instructions, about 3•5 minutes.

3. Remove from heat and ladle the Fukuoka style ramen into bowls.

4. Top each serving with slices of pork belly or chashu pork, soft boiled egg halves, bean sprouts, and sliced green onions.

5. Serve hot, with pickled ginger on the side if desired.

The key features of Fukuoka style ramen are the rich, pork bone•based broth and the thinly sliced pork belly or chashu pork topping. The soy sauce, mirin, and white pepper create a savory, slightly sweet, and peppery flavor profile. The soft boiled egg, bean sprouts, and green onions add freshness and texture.

This style of ramen originates from the Fukuoka prefecture in Japan, known for its delicious pork•based dishes. The long•simmered pork bone broth gives this ramen a deep, complex flavor that is truly authentic to the Fukuoka region.

97. Hakata Style Ramen

Ingredient:

- 8 oz thin, straight ramen noodles
- 4 cups pork bone broth
- 2 tbsp soy sauce
- 1 tbsp sesame oil
- 1 tsp white sugar
- 1/2 tsp ground white pepper

- 1 cup thinly sliced pork belly or chashu pork
- 2 soft boiled eggs, halved
- 1 cup bean sprouts
- 2 green onions, sliced
- Pickled ginger for serving (optional)

Instructions:

1. In a large pot, combine the pork bone broth, soy sauce, sesame oil, sugar, and white pepper. Bring to a simmer over medium heat.

2. Add the thin, straight ramen noodles to the pot and cook according to package instructions, about 2•3 minutes.

3. Remove from heat and ladle the Hakata style ramen into bowls.

4. Top each serving with slices of pork belly or chashu pork, soft boiled egg halves, bean sprouts, and sliced green onions.

5. Serve hot, with pickled ginger on the side if desired.

The hallmarks of Hakata style ramen are the use of a rich, pork bone•based broth and thin, straight ramen noodles. The broth is seasoned simply with soy sauce, sesame oil, sugar, and white pepper, allowing the pork flavor to shine.

The thinly sliced pork belly or chashu pork, soft boiled egg, bean sprouts, and green onions are classic Hakata•style toppings that add texture and freshness to balance the hearty broth.

This style of ramen originates from the Hakata district of Fukuoka city in Kyushu, Japan, known for its exceptional ramen shops. The focus is on the quality of the broth and noodles, resulting in a pure, refined flavor profile.

This Hakata style ramen would be an excellent option for those looking to experience an authentic, traditional Japanese ramen dish. The simple yet delicious flavors make it a satisfying and comforting meal.

98. Nagoya Style Ramen

Ingredient:

• 8 oz ramen noodles
• 4 cups chicken or pork broth
• 2 tbsp miso paste
• 1 tbsp soy sauce
• 1 tsp sesame oil
• 1 tsp sugar
• 1/2 tsp ground black pepper
• 1 cup shredded pork or chicken
• 2 soft boiled eggs, halved
• 1 cup shredded cabbage
• 2 green onions, sliced
• 1 sheet of nori, cut into strips
• Toasted sesame seeds for garnish

Instructions:

1. In a large pot, bring the broth to a simmer over medium heat. Whisk in the miso paste, soy sauce, sesame oil, sugar, and black pepper until fully incorporated.

2. Add the ramen noodles to the pot and cook according to package instructions, about 3•5 minutes.

3. Stir in the shredded pork or chicken and cook for an additional 2•3 minutes until heated through.

4. Remove from heat and ladle the Nagoya style ramen into bowls.

5. Top each serving with a soft boiled egg half, shredded cabbage, sliced green onions, nori strips, and a sprinkle of toasted sesame seeds.

6. Serve hot and enjoy the bold, savory flavors of this Nagoya•inspired ramen!

The key elements of Nagoya style ramen are the use of miso paste, soy sauce, and sesame oil to create a rich, umami•forward broth. The addition of shredded pork or chicken provides heartiness, while the soft boiled egg, cabbage, and nori add texture and freshness. This ramen has a bold, slightly spicy flavor profile that is signature to the Nagoya region of Japan.

99. Hiroshima Style Ramen

Ingredient:

• 8 oz fresh ramen noodles
• 4 cups chicken or vegetable broth
• 2 tbsp soy sauce
• 1 tsp sesame oil
• 2 cups thinly sliced cabbage
• 1 carrot, julienned
• 2 green onions, sliced
• 2 eggs, soft boiled
• Sriracha or other hot sauce (optional)

Instructions:

1. Bring the broth, soy sauce, and sesame oil to a simmer in a large pot. Add the ramen noodles and cook for 2•3 minutes until tender.

2. Add the sliced cabbage and julienned carrot to the pot. Cook for 1•2 minutes until the vegetables are slightly softened.

3. Carefully add the soft boiled eggs to the pot.

4. Remove from heat and stir in the green onions.

5. Divide the ramen between 2•4 bowls. Serve immediately, with Sriracha or other hot sauce on the side if desired.

The key features of Hiroshima•style ramen are the addition of cabbage and carrot, which add texture and crunch, as well as the soft boiled egg. The broth is light and flavorful, allowing the other ingredients to shine. Feel free to adjust the vegetable amounts to your preference. Enjoy this delicious regional ramen variation!

100. Okinawa Style Ramen

Ingredient:

- 8 oz ramen noodles
- 4 cups pork or chicken broth
- 2 tbsp soy sauce
- 1 tbsp mirin
- 1 tsp sesame oil
- 1/2 tsp ground black pepper
- 1 cup sliced char siu pork
- 1 cup shredded cabbage
- 1 cup bean sprouts
- 2 green onions, sliced
- 1 soft boiled egg, halved
- Pickled red ginger for serving (optional)

Instructions:

1. In a large pot, combine the broth, soy sauce, mirin, sesame oil, and black pepper. Bring to a simmer over medium heat.

2. Add the ramen noodles to the pot and cook according to package instructions, about 3-5 minutes.

3. Remove from heat and stir in the sliced char siu pork, shredded cabbage, and bean sprouts.

4. Ladle the Okinawa style ramen into bowls.

5. Top each serving with a soft boiled egg half, sliced green onions, and a side of pickled red ginger, if desired. Serve hot and enjoy the bold, savory flavors of this Okinawan-inspired ramen.

Okinawa, the southernmost prefecture of Japan, has its own unique take on ramen that reflects the island's subtropical climate and culinary influences. This style features a pork or chicken-based broth seasoned with soy sauce, mirin, and black pepper.

The toppings of char siu pork, cabbage, bean sprouts, and soft boiled egg provide a variety of textures and flavors. The pickled red ginger is an optional garnish that adds a bright, tangy contrast.

This Okinawa style ramen would be a great option for those looking to explore the diverse regional styles of Japanese ramen. The bold, savory broth and hearty toppings make it a satisfying and comforting meal. Adjust the seasoning to your taste preferences.

101. Chicken and Egg Ramen

Ingredient:

• 8 oz ramen noodles
• 4 cups chicken broth
• 2 tbsp soy sauce
• 1 tsp sesame oil
• 1 lb boneless, skinless chicken thighs, cut into bite•sized pieces
• 2 eggs, soft boiled
• 2 green onions, sliced
• 2 cups baby spinach
• Salt and pepper to taste

Instructions:

1. Bring the chicken broth, soy sauce, and sesame oil to a simmer in a large pot. Add the ramen noodles and cook for 2•3 minutes until tender.

2. Add the chicken pieces to the pot and cook for 3•4 minutes until cooked through.

3. Carefully add the soft boiled eggs to the pot.

4. Remove from heat and stir in the green onions and baby spinach. Season with salt and pepper to taste.

5. Divide the ramen between 2•4 bowls and serve immediately.

The soft boiled eggs add a rich, creamy element to the broth, while the chicken provides protein. The spinach and green onions add freshness. Adjust any seasonings to your liking. Enjoy your homemade Chicken and Egg Ramen!

102. Steak and Egg Ramen

Ingredient:

• 8 oz ramen noodles
• 4 cups beef or chicken broth
• 2 tbsp soy sauce
• 1 tsp sesame oil
• 8 oz thinly sliced steak (such as flank or skirt steak)
• 2 eggs, soft boiled
• 2 green onions, sliced
• 2 cups baby spinach
• Salt and pepper to taste

Instructions:

1. Bring the broth, soy sauce, and sesame oil to a simmer in a large pot. Add the ramen noodles and cook for 2•3 minutes until tender.

2. Add the sliced steak to the pot and cook for 1•2 minutes until just cooked through.

3. Carefully add the soft boiled eggs to the pot.

4. Remove from heat and stir in the green onions and baby spinach. Season with salt and pepper to taste.

5. Divide the ramen between 2•4 bowls and serve immediately.

The soft boiled eggs add a rich, creamy element to the broth, while the steak provides protein. The spinach and green onions add freshness. Adjust any seasonings to your liking. Enjoy your homemade Steak and Egg Ramen!

103. Shrimp and Egg Ramen

Ingredient:

- 8 oz ramen noodles
- 4 cups chicken or vegetable broth
- 2 tbsp soy sauce
- 1 tsp sesame oil
- 1 lb shrimp, peeled and deveined
- 2 eggs, soft boiled
- 2 green onions, sliced
- 2 cups baby spinach
- Salt and pepper to taste

Instructions:

1. Bring the broth, soy sauce, and sesame oil to a simmer in a large pot. Add the ramen noodles and cook for 2•3 minutes until tender.

2. Add the shrimp to the pot and cook for 2•3 minutes until they turn pink and opaque.

3. Carefully add the soft boiled eggs to the pot.

4. Remove from heat and stir in the green onions and baby spinach. Season with salt and pepper to taste.

5. Divide the ramen between 2•4 bowls and serve immediately.

The soft boiled eggs add a rich, creamy element to the broth, while the shrimp provides protein. The spinach and green onions add freshness. Adjust any seasonings to your liking. Enjoy your homemade Shrimp and Egg Ramen!

104. Tofu and Egg Ramen

Ingredient:

- 8 oz ramen noodles
- 4 cups chicken or vegetable broth
- 2 tbsp soy sauce
- 1 tsp sesame oil
- 1 block firm tofu, cubed
- 2 eggs, soft boiled
- 2 green onions, sliced
- 2 cups baby spinach
- Salt and pepper to taste

Instructions:

1. Bring the broth, soy sauce, and sesame oil to a simmer in a large pot. Add the ramen noodles and cook for 2•3 minutes until tender.

2. Gently add the cubed tofu and cook for 1•2 minutes until heated through.

3. Carefully add the soft boiled eggs to the pot.

4. Remove from heat and stir in the green onions and baby spinach. Season with salt and pepper to taste.

5. Divide the ramen between 2•4 bowls and serve immediately.

The soft boiled eggs add a rich, creamy element to the broth, while the tofu provides protein. The spinach and green onions add freshness. Adjust any seasonings to your liking. Enjoy your homemade Tofu and Egg Ramen!

105. Salmon Ramen

Ingredient:

• 8 oz ramen noodles
• 4 cups chicken or vegetable broth
• 2 tbsp soy sauce
• 1 tsp sesame oil
• 8 oz salmon fillets, cut into bite•sized pieces
• 2 eggs, soft boiled
• 2 green onions, sliced
• 2 cups baby spinach
• Salt and pepper to taste

Instructions:

1. Bring the broth, soy sauce, and sesame oil to a simmer in a large pot. Add the ramen noodles and cook for 2•3 minutes until tender.

2. Add the salmon pieces to the pot and cook for 2•3 minutes until just cooked through.

3. Carefully add the soft boiled eggs to the pot.

4. Remove from heat and stir in the green onions and baby spinach. Season with salt and pepper to taste.

5. Divide the ramen between 2•4 bowls and serve immediately.

The salmon adds a delicious, healthy protein to the ramen, while the soft boiled eggs provide richness. The spinach and green onions add freshness. You can use fresh or canned salmon. Adjust any seasonings to your liking. Enjoy your Salmon Ramen!

106. Crab Ramen

Ingredient:

- 8 oz ramen noodles
- 4 cups seafood or chicken broth
- 2 tbsp soy sauce
- 1 tsp sesame oil
- 8 oz lump crab meat, picked over for shells
- 2 eggs, soft boiled
- 2 green onions, sliced
- 2 cups baby spinach
- Salt and pepper to taste

Instructions:

1. Bring the broth, soy sauce, and sesame oil to a simmer in a large pot. Add the ramen noodles and cook for 2·3 minutes until tender.

2. Gently stir in the crab meat and cook for 1·2 minutes until heated through.

3. Carefully add the soft boiled eggs to the pot.

4. Remove from heat and stir in the green onions and baby spinach. Season with salt and pepper to taste.

5. Divide the ramen between 2·4 bowls and serve immediately.

The crab meat adds a sweet, delicate seafood flavor to the broth, while the soft boiled eggs provide richness. The spinach and green onions add freshness. You can use lump crab or shredded crab meat. Adjust any seasonings to your liking. Enjoy your Crab Ramen!

107. Lamb Ramen

Ingredient:

• 8 oz ramen noodles
• 4 cups beef or chicken broth
• 2 tbsp soy sauce
• 1 tsp sesame oil
• 8 oz ground lamb
• 2 eggs, soft boiled
• 2 green onions, sliced
• 2 cups baby spinach
• Salt and pepper to taste

Instructions:

1. Bring the broth, soy sauce, and sesame oil to a simmer in a large pot. Add the ramen noodles and cook for 2•3 minutes until tender.

2. Add the ground lamb to the pot and cook, breaking it up with a spoon, for 3•4 minutes until browned and cooked through.

3. Carefully add the soft boiled eggs to the pot.

4. Remove from heat and stir in the green onions and baby spinach. Season with salt and pepper to taste.

5. Divide the ramen between 2•4 bowls and serve immediately.

The ground lamb adds a rich, savory flavor to the ramen broth. The soft boiled eggs provide creaminess, while the spinach and green onions add freshness. You can use ground lamb or lamb sausage meat. Adjust any seasonings to your preference. Enjoy this hearty Lamb Ramen!

108. Venison Ramen

Ingredient:

• 8 oz ramen noodles
• 4 cups beef or chicken broth
• 2 tbsp soy sauce
• 1 tsp sesame oil
• 8 oz ground venison
• 2 eggs, soft boiled
• 2 green onions, sliced
• 2 cups baby spinach
• Salt and pepper to taste

Instructions:

1. Bring the broth, soy sauce, and sesame oil to a simmer in a large pot. Add the ramen noodles and cook for 2•3 minutes until tender.

2. Add the ground venison to the pot and cook, breaking it up with a spoon, for 3•4 minutes until browned and cooked through.

3. Carefully add the soft boiled eggs to the pot.

4. Remove from heat and stir in the green onions and baby spinach. Season with salt and pepper to taste.

5. Divide the ramen between 2•4 bowls and serve immediately.

The ground venison adds a rich, gamey flavor to the ramen broth. The soft boiled eggs provide creaminess, while the spinach and green onions add freshness. You can use ground venison or venison sausage meat. Adjust any seasonings to your preference. Enjoy this hearty Venison Ramen!

109. Turkey Ramen

Ingredient:

- 8 oz ramen noodles
- 4 cups turkey or chicken broth
- 2 tbsp soy sauce
- 1 tbsp mirin
- 1 tsp sesame oil
- 1/2 tsp ground ginger
- 1/4 tsp white pepper
- 2 cups shredded cooked turkey
- 1 cup shredded cabbage
- 1 cup sliced mushrooms
- 2 green onions, sliced
- 2 soft boiled eggs, halved (optional)
- Chopped cilantro for garnish

Instructions:

1. In a large pot, combine the turkey or chicken broth, soy sauce, mirin, sesame oil, ground ginger, and white pepper. Bring to a simmer over medium heat.

2. Add the ramen noodles to the pot and cook according to package instructions, about 3•5 minutes.

3. Stir in the shredded cooked turkey, shredded cabbage, and sliced mushrooms. Cook for an additional 2•3 minutes until the vegetables are tender.

4. Remove from heat and ladle the turkey ramen into bowls.

5. Top each serving with a soft boiled egg half (if using), sliced green onions, and chopped cilantro. Serve hot and enjoy this comforting turkey•based ramen.

This turkey ramen is a great way to use up leftover turkey, whether from Thanksgiving or any other roasted turkey meal. The turkey broth provides a rich, savory base, while the soy sauce, mirin, and spices add depth of flavor.

The shredded turkey, cabbage, and mushrooms give the ramen heartiness and texture. The soft boiled egg is an optional addition that adds creaminess. The fresh cilantro garnish brightens up the dish.

This turkey ramen would be a delicious and creative way to enjoy the flavors of Thanksgiving in a comforting ramen bowl. It's a great option for teens or anyone looking for a unique twist on classic ramen.

110. Ham Ramen

Ingredient:

- 4 cups chicken or vegetable broth
- 2 tablespoons soy sauce
- 1 tablespoon rice vinegar
- 1 teaspoon sesame oil
- 1/2 teaspoon ground ginger
- 2 packages ramen noodles (discard seasoning packets)
- 1 cup shredded cooked ham
- 2 cups shredded cabbage or spinach
- 2 green onions, sliced
- 2 soft•boiled eggs (optional)

Instructions:

1. In a large pot, bring the broth, soy sauce, rice vinegar, sesame oil, and ground ginger to a simmer over medium heat.

2. Add the ramen noodles and cook for 2•3 minutes, until tender.

3. Stir in the shredded ham, cabbage/spinach, and green onions. Cook for 1•2 minutes more, until the greens are wilted.

4. Ladle the ramen into bowls. Top each serving with a soft•boiled egg, if desired.

5. Serve hot and enjoy!

The combination of savory ham, crunchy vegetables, and soft ramen noodles in a flavorful broth makes this ham ramen a delicious and satisfying meal. Feel free to adjust the ingredients to your taste preferences.

111. Cinnamon Sugar Ramen

Ingredient:

• 2 packages ramen noodles (discard seasoning packets)
• 2 cups milk
• 2 tablespoons brown sugar
• 1 teaspoon ground cinnamon
• 1/4 teaspoon ground nutmeg
• 1 tablespoon butter
• Whipped cream (optional)
• Chopped toasted pecans (optional)

Instructions:

1. Bring a pot of water to a boil. Add the ramen noodles and cook according to package instructions, about 3 minutes. Drain and set aside.

2. In a medium saucepan, whisk together the milk, brown sugar, cinnamon, and nutmeg. Heat over medium, stirring frequently, until the mixture is warm and the sugar has dissolved, about 5 minutes.

3. Remove the saucepan from the heat and stir in the butter until melted and fully incorporated.

4. Add the cooked ramen noodles to the cinnamon•sugar milk mixture and toss to coat the noodles evenly.

5. Serve the cinnamon sugar ramen warm, topped with a dollop of whipped cream and a sprinkle of chopped toasted pecans, if desired.

The creamy, sweet, and spiced cinnamon sugar sauce coats the ramen noodles, creating a comforting and indulgent breakfast or dessert•like dish. Adjust the amounts of sugar and spices to your taste preferences.

112. Caramel Ramen

Ingredient:

• 2 packages ramen noodles (discard seasoning packets)
• 1/2 cup brown sugar
• 1/4 cup butter
• 2 tablespoons heavy cream
• 1/2 teaspoon vanilla extract
• 1/4 teaspoon salt
• Whipped cream (optional)
• Chopped toasted pecans (optional)

Instructions:

1. Bring a pot of water to a boil. Add the ramen noodles and cook according to package instructions, about 3 minutes. Drain and set aside.

2. In a medium saucepan, combine the brown sugar, butter, heavy cream, vanilla extract, and salt. Cook over medium heat, stirring constantly, until the mixture comes to a boil and thickens, about 5•7 minutes.

3. Remove the saucepan from the heat and carefully pour the caramel sauce over the cooked ramen noodles. Toss the noodles to coat them evenly in the caramel.

4. Serve the caramel ramen warm, topped with a dollop of whipped cream and a sprinkle of chopped toasted pecans, if desired.

The rich, gooey caramel sauce coats the ramen noodles, creating a decadent and indulgent dish. The combination of the sweet caramel, creamy noodles, and crunchy pecans makes for a delightful treat.

Adjust the amount of brown sugar and cream to your desired level of sweetness and consistency. You can also experiment with different toppings, such as crushed graham crackers or a drizzle of chocolate sauce.

113. Apple Pie Ramen

Ingredient:

• 2 packages ramen noodles (discard seasoning packets)
• 2 cups peeled and diced apples (about 2 medium apples)
• 1/4 cup brown sugar
• 1 teaspoon ground cinnamon
• 1/4 teaspoon ground nutmeg
• 2 tablespoons butter
• 1/4 cup heavy cream
• Whipped cream (optional)
• Crushed graham crackers (optional)

Instructions:

1. Bring a pot of water to a boil. Add the ramen noodles and cook according to package instructions, about 3 minutes. Drain and set aside.

2. In a medium saucepan, combine the diced apples, brown sugar, cinnamon, and nutmeg. Cook over medium heat, stirring occasionally, until the apples are softened and the mixture is bubbly, about 8•10 minutes.

3. Remove the saucepan from the heat and stir in the butter and heavy cream until the butter is melted and the mixture is well combined.

4. Add the cooked ramen noodles to the apple mixture and toss to coat the noodles evenly.

5. Serve the apple pie ramen warm, topped with a dollop of whipped cream and a sprinkle of crushed graham crackers, if desired.

The sweet and spiced apple mixture coats the ramen noodles, creating a comforting and dessert•like dish. The combination of the soft, tender apples, creamy noodles, and crunchy graham crackers makes for a delightful and unique twist on traditional ramen.

Adjust the amount of sugar and spices to your taste preferences. You can also experiment with different types of apples or add a splash of vanilla extract for additional flavor.

114. Pumpkin Pie Ramen

Ingredient:

• 2 packages ramen noodles (discard seasoning packets)
• 1 cup canned pumpkin puree
• 1/2 cup heavy cream
• 1/4 cup brown sugar
• 1 teaspoon ground cinnamon
• 1/2 teaspoon ground ginger
• 1/4 teaspoon ground nutmeg
• 1/4 teaspoon salt
• Whipped cream (optional)
• Crushed graham crackers (optional)

Instructions:

1. Bring a pot of water to a boil. Add the ramen noodles and cook according to package instructions, about 3 minutes. Drain and set aside.

2. In a medium saucepan, whisk together the pumpkin puree, heavy cream, brown sugar, cinnamon, ginger, nutmeg, and salt. Cook over medium heat, stirring frequently, until the mixture is warm and the sugar has dissolved, about 5•7 minutes.

3. Remove the saucepan from the heat and add the cooked ramen noodles. Toss the noodles to coat them evenly in the pumpkin mixture.

4. Serve the pumpkin pie ramen warm, topped with a dollop of whipped cream and a sprinkle of crushed graham crackers, if desired.

The creamy, spiced pumpkin sauce coats the ramen noodles, creating a comforting and dessert•like dish. The combination of the rich pumpkin, warm spices, and crunchy graham crackers makes for a delightful and unique twist on traditional ramen.

Adjust the amount of sugar and spices to your taste preferences. You can also experiment with different toppings, such as toasted pecans or a drizzle of caramel sauce.

115. S'mores Ramen

Ingredient:

• 2 packages ramen noodles (discard seasoning packets)
• 2 cups milk
• 1/4 cup granulated sugar
• 2 tablespoons unsweetened cocoa powder
• 1/2 teaspoon vanilla extract
• 1 cup miniature marshmallows
• 1/2 cup crushed graham crackers
• Chocolate syrup (optional)

Instructions:

1. Bring a pot of water to a boil. Add the ramen noodles and cook according to package instructions, about 3 minutes. Drain and set aside.

2. In a medium saucepan, whisk together the milk, sugar, and cocoa powder. Cook over medium heat, stirring frequently, until the mixture is warm and the sugar has dissolved, about 5 minutes.

3. Remove the saucepan from the heat and stir in the vanilla extract.

4. Add the cooked ramen noodles to the chocolate milk mixture and toss to coat the noodles evenly.

5. Divide the s'mores ramen into serving bowls and top with the miniature marshmallows and crushed graham crackers.

6. Drizzle with chocolate syrup, if desired.

7. Serve the s'mores ramen warm and enjoy!

The rich, chocolatey ramen noodles are topped with gooey marshmallows and crunchy graham crackers, creating a delightful and indulgent twist on the classic s'mores flavor. The combination of the soft, creamy noodles and the sweet, toasted toppings makes for a truly unique and satisfying dish.

Adjust the amount of sugar and cocoa powder to your desired level of sweetness. You can also experiment with different toppings, such as chopped nuts or a sprinkle of cinnamon.

116. Chocolate Mint Ramen

Ingredient:

• 2 packages ramen noodles (discard seasoning packets)
• 2 cups milk
• 1/4 cup granulated sugar
• 2 tablespoons unsweetened cocoa powder
• 1/2 teaspoon peppermint extract
• 1/4 teaspoon salt
• Whipped cream (optional)
• Crushed peppermint candies (optional)

Instructions:

1. Bring a pot of water to a boil. Add the ramen noodles and cook according to package instructions, about 3 minutes. Drain and set aside.

2. In a medium saucepan, whisk together the milk, sugar, cocoa powder, peppermint extract, and salt. Cook over medium heat, stirring frequently, until the mixture is warm and the sugar has dissolved, about 5 minutes.

3. Remove the saucepan from the heat and add the cooked ramen noodles. Toss the noodles to coat them evenly in the chocolate mint mixture.

4. Serve the chocolate mint ramen warm, topped with a dollop of whipped cream and a sprinkle of crushed peppermint candies, if desired.

The rich, chocolatey ramen noodles are infused with a refreshing peppermint flavor, creating a unique and indulgent twist on traditional ramen. The combination of the creamy, minty sauce and the soft, chewy noodles makes for a delightful and comforting dish.

Adjust the amount of peppermint extract to your desired level of minty flavor. You can also experiment with different toppings, such as shaved dark chocolate or a drizzle of caramel sauce.

117. Banana Split Ramen

Ingredient:

• 2 packages ramen noodles (discard seasoning packets)
• 2 ripe bananas, sliced
• 1/2 cup chocolate syrup
• 1/2 cup strawberry syrup
• 1 cup vanilla ice cream
• Whipped cream
• Maraschino cherries
• Chopped toasted nuts (optional)

Instructions:

1. Bring a pot of water to a boil. Add the ramen noodles and cook according to package instructions, about 3 minutes. Drain and set aside.

2. In a large bowl, combine the cooked ramen noodles and sliced bananas.

3. Drizzle the chocolate syrup and strawberry syrup over the noodles and bananas, gently tossing to coat.

4. Scoop the vanilla ice cream into the center of the ramen and banana mixture.

5. Top the dish with whipped cream, maraschino cherries, and chopped toasted nuts (if using).

6. Serve the banana split ramen immediately, while the ice cream is still frozen.

The combination of the soft, chewy ramen noodles, sweet bananas, rich chocolate and strawberry syrups, and creamy vanilla ice cream creates a unique and indulgent twist on the classic banana split. The whipped cream and cherries add a touch of elegance, while the optional nuts provide a crunchy contrast.

Feel free to adjust the amounts of syrups and toppings to your personal taste preferences. You can also experiment with different ice cream flavors or add other fruit, such as sliced strawberries or pineapple.

118. Red Velvet Ramen

Ingredient:

• 2 packages ramen noodles (discard seasoning packets)
• 2 cups milk
• 1/4 cup granulated sugar
• 2 tablespoons unsweetened cocoa powder
• 1 tablespoon red food coloring
• 1 teaspoon vanilla extract
• 1/4 teaspoon salt
• Cream cheese frosting (optional)
• Crushed Oreos or chocolate wafers (optional)

Instructions:

1. Bring a pot of water to a boil. Add the ramen noodles and cook according to package instructions, about 3 minutes. Drain and set aside.

2. In a medium saucepan, whisk together the milk, sugar, cocoa powder, red food coloring, vanilla extract, and salt. Cook over medium heat, stirring frequently, until the mixture is warm and the sugar has dissolved, about 5 minutes.

3. Remove the saucepan from the heat and add the cooked ramen noodles. Toss the noodles to coat them evenly in the red velvet mixture.

4. Serve the red velvet ramen warm, topped with a dollop of cream cheese frosting and a sprinkle of crushed Oreos or chocolate wafers, if desired.

The rich, chocolatey ramen noodles are infused with a vibrant red color and a hint of vanilla, creating a unique and indulgent twist on traditional ramen. The creamy frosting and crunchy cookie topping add a delightful contrast in texture and flavor.

Adjust the amount of food coloring to achieve your desired shade of red. You can also experiment with different toppings, such as toasted coconut, chopped nuts, or a drizzle of white chocolate.

119. Lemon Meringue Ramen

Ingredient:

• 2 packages ramen noodles (discard seasoning packets)
• 1 cup milk
• 1/4 cup granulated sugar
• 2 tablespoons lemon juice
• 1 teaspoon lemon zest
• 2 egg whites
• 1/4 cup powdered sugar
• Toasted meringue topping (optional)

Instructions:

1. Bring a pot of water to a boil. Add the ramen noodles and cook according to package instructions, about 3 minutes. Drain and set aside.

2. In a medium saucepan, whisk together the milk, granulated sugar, lemon juice, and lemon zest. Cook over medium heat, stirring frequently, until the mixture is warm and the sugar has dissolved, about 5 minutes.

3. Remove the saucepan from the heat and add the cooked ramen noodles. Toss the noodles to coat them evenly in the lemon mixture.

4. In a separate bowl, beat the egg whites with an electric mixer until they form soft peaks. Gradually add the powdered sugar and continue beating until the meringue is stiff and glossy.

5. Serve the lemon meringue ramen warm, topped with the toasted meringue topping, if desired.

The bright, tangy lemon flavor of the ramen noodles is complemented by the sweet, fluffy meringue topping, creating a unique and refreshing twist on traditional ramen. The combination of the soft, chewy noodles and the light, airy meringue makes for a delightful and indulgent dish.

Adjust the amount of lemon juice and zest to your desired level of tartness. You can also experiment with different toppings, such as a drizzle of lemon curd or a sprinkle of toasted coconut.

Congratulations on completing *Ramen Cookbook for Teens: 115+ Homemade Ramen Favorites Every Teen Can Cook.* We hope this cookbook has sparked your passion for cooking and empowered you to create delicious and satisfying ramen dishes right in your own kitchen. Whether you're new to cooking or already an enthusiastic chef, mastering the art of homemade ramen opens up a world of culinary possibilities.

Reflecting on Your Journey

Throughout this cookbook, you've explored over 115 recipes that showcase the diversity and creativity of ramen. From classic flavors to innovative twists, each recipe was crafted with teens in mind—emphasizing simplicity, ease of preparation, and, most importantly, great taste.

Key Takeaways

As you continue your culinary journey, here are some key takeaways to remember:

- *Cooking is an Adventure:* Embrace the joy of experimenting with flavors and ingredients to create your own unique ramen creations.

- *Skills and Confidence:* Building cooking skills not only enhances your abilities in the kitchen but also boosts your confidence in trying new recipes and techniques.

- *Healthier Choices:* Homemade ramen allows you to control ingredients, making it easier to create nutritious and balanced meals.

- *Sharing with Others:* Share your love of cooking by preparing delicious meals for family and friends, creating memorable experiences around the dinner table.

Embrace Your Creativity

Cooking is a form of self-expression and creativity. Don't be afraid to customize recipes, swap ingredients, or add your own flair to make each dish uniquely yours. The possibilities with ramen are endless, so continue to explore, experiment, and enjoy the process of creating meals that bring joy and satisfaction.

Final Thoughts

Thank you for joining us on this flavorful journey through homemade ramen. We hope this cookbook has inspired you to continue exploring new cuisines, trying different recipes, and expanding your culinary horizons. Remember, cooking is a lifelong skill that brings joy, nourishment, and connection to others.